Advanced Pathology and Treatment of Diseases of Poultry

With Special Reference to Etiology, Signs, Pathology and Management

C.D.N. Singh
B.V.Sc & A.H., M.Sc (Vet.), Gold medalist, Ph. D.,F.R.V.C.S (Sweden)
Formerly University Professor-cum-Chairman of Pathology,
Bihar Veterinary College, Patna, INDIA

S.D. Singh
B.V.Sc. & A.H., M.V.Sc., Ph.D.
Formerly Associate Professor of Pharmacology, Ex-Principal
Bihar Veterinary College, Patna, INDIA

S.P. Verma
B.V.Sc. & A.H., M.V.Sc., Ph.D.
Principal
Bihar Veterinary College, Patna, INDIA

L.N.Prasad
B.V.Sc. & A.H., M.V.Sc., Ph.D.
Formerly Associate Professor of Pathology,
Bihar Veterinary College, Patna, INDIA

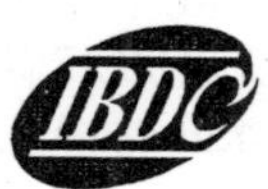

International Book Distributing Co.
(Publishing Division)

Published by

INTERNATIONAL BOOK DISTRIBUTING CO.

(Publishing Division)
Chaman Studio Building, 2nd Floor,
Charbagh, Lucknow 226 004 U.P. (INDIA)
Tel. : Off. : 2450004, 2450007, 2459058 Fax : 0522-2458629
E-Mail : ibdco@sancharnet.in

First Edition 2006

MAXIMUM RETAIL PRICE INCLUSIVE OF ALL TAXES Rs 725.00

Price: (B)
ISBN 81-8189-167-8

Composed & Designed at :

Panacea Computers
3rd Floor, Agrawal Sabha Bhawan
Subhash Mohal, Sadar Cantt. Lucknow-226 00
Phone : 0522-2483312, 9335927082
E-mail : prasgupt@rediffmail.com

Printed at:

Salasar Imaging Systems
C-7/5, Lawrence Road Industrial Area
Delhi - 110 035
Tel. : 011-27185653, 9810064311

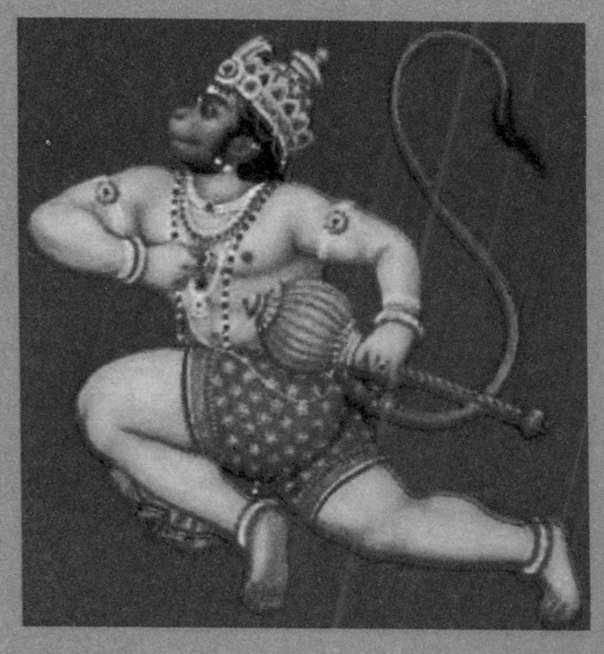

Dedicated
to
Lord Pawansut Hanuman ji
and
to the memory of late Vina Singh,
wife of the first author

Foreword

I have much pleasure to introduce this book to students and teachers in the subject of poultry diseases and their treatment. The two subjects of pathology and medicine have been combined into one in a very easy and lucid language. This book presents useful coverage of signs and lesions of poultry diseases with special emphasis on their treatment.

I congratulate Dr. C.D.N. Singh, Dr. S.D.Singh, Dr. S. P. Verma and Dr. L.N. Prasad [the co-authors] for the magnificent presentation they have done.

SITA RAM SINGH
Vice-Chancellor, R.A.U.
Bihar, Pusa (Samastipur)

संदेश

डॉ सी.डी.एन. सिंह, भूतपूर्व विश्वविद्यालय प्राध्यापक, बिहार वेटनरी कॉलेज, पटना एवं सह-लेखकों द्वारा लिखित पुस्तक 'Advanced Pathology and Treatment of Diseases of Poultry' का प्रथम संस्करण के प्रकाशन की बात जानकर मुझे अपार हर्ष हो रहा है। कुकुट पालन उद्योग भारत वर्ष में मजबूत जड़ बना चुका है, जिससे समाज का बहुत बड़ा गरीब तबका इस उद्योग से जुड़ा हुआ है। कुकुटों की बीमारी के रोक-थाम एवं उपचार हेतु पुस्तक लेखन का यह प्रयास सराहनीय है। आशा है कि इस पुस्तक से छात्र, पशु चिकित्सक एवं मुर्गी पालक लाभान्वित होंगे। राजेन्द्र कृषि विश्वविद्यालय पूसा, समस्तीपुर शिक्षा, शोध, प्रसार एवं पुस्तक लेखन तथा जन साधारण के लिए उपयोगी शोध आधारित तकनीकी प्रकाशन आदि विकास कार्य का समय बंध दायित्व पालन करता रहेगा।

नरेन्द्र सिंह
कृषि मंत्री, कृषि विभाग
बिहार सरकार, पटना

Message

Dr. C.D.N. Singh, former University Professor of Veterinary Pathology, Bihar Veterinary College, Patna, is a well known scientist cum teacher in the field of Veterinary Pathology. His teaching, research and field extension programmes had made a distinct mark amongst the veterinary students, animal and poultry farmers. I am happy to see that his wide experience and knowledge is now taking shape in the form of a book entitled 'Advanced Pathology and Treatment of diseases of Poultry' which is so badly needed in the modern science and technology for better results. I have gone through the various chapters which provide deep insight into the scientific understanding of the problems. This publication is all the more important in view of the current poultry diseases like bird flue affecting the whole world. I hope this publication would benefit all concerned and I congratulate the author Dr. Singh for this endeavour.

17-04-2006

Prof. (Dr.) Gopal Trivedi
B.Sc. (Ag.), M.Sc. (Ag.), Ph.D.
Ex-Vice Chancellor, RAU, Pusa (Bihar)

PREFACE

The book 'Advanced pathology and treatment of diseases of poultry' has been prepared to cater to the needs of students of the veterinary colleges, diagnosticians engaged in disease investigations and practicing veterinarians in different states of this country. The syllabi prevalent in different agricultural universities have been kept in view in preparing the manuscript of this book. We have inserted all pertinent pathological changes in different poultry diseases with the object of making this book of high value to the students at both undergraduate and postgraduate levels in the veterinary colleges. More and more stress has been laid on the information in relation to signs, gross and microscopic lesions of avain diseases prevalent in poultry flock for their quick diagnoses. We are grateful to pathologists like Professor P.B. Kuppuswamy, Bihar Veterinary College, Patna, Professor S.Rubarth, Royal Veterinary College Stockholm, Sweden and various scholars whose views have been included in this book. Thanks are also due to Anima Kumari, Kankarbagh, Patna for carefully typing out the manuscript of this book.

Thanks are due to Dr. Satya Vrat Singh, Assistant Professor, College of Veterinary Sciences, NDUA&T, Faizabad for his valued advice in preparing the manuscript of the text.

We lay no claim to any originalities and welcome suggestions and healthy criticisms of the subject matter for further improvement of this book.

C.D.N.Singh
S.D.Singh
S.P.Verma
L.N.Prasad

Contents

1

Poultry Diseases

The cellular reactions of the birds to the various kinds of noxious agents like bacteria, viruses, protozoa and mineral deprivations are almost similar to those in the mammalian tissues. There may be some minor differences due to species or other biological factors e.g. calcification is not a feature of tuberculous lesions in fowls. Acute exudative inflammatory reactions are noticed in Newcastle disease, infectious laryngotracheitis, coryza and coccidiosis but the chronic granulomatous lesions are the marked changes in aspergillosis, tuberculosis and coligranuloma. Certain diseases are noticed in very acute form in some age groups of birds as exemplified in Gumboro disease (chickens, aged 3-6 weeks) and Marek's disease (chickens aged 3-9 weeks). Degenerative (necrotic) changes in the lymphoid cells of cloacal bursa in infectious bursal disease (IBD), haemorrhagic-necrotic intestinal lesions in RD (Ranikhet disease) and coagulation necrosis, heterophil accumulation, hyperplasia of synovial cells, lymphocytes, macrophages and plasma cells in viral arthritis in birds are important features of the disease processes .

Diseases in the poultry result from impairment of body functions. Proper sanitation is of utmost importance in prevention and control of poultry diseases. Stresses of different kinds (chills, overexhaustion and starvation etc.) render the chickens susceptible to diseases. The factors controlling the occurrence of diseases are as under:

[1] Number of birds

[2] Types of birds

[3] Virulence (the ability to produce diseases) of the pathogens

[4] Route of entry

[5] Biological factors like defense status or capability

Mild round worm infection in the poultry is not a serious problem. Several infectious organisms cause heavy mortality or moribund state in the flocks of birds. Many poultry diseases can be controlled by following the fundamental management procedures. A good breeding policy has helped development of the birds resistant to many infectious diseases. Feeds of good quality protect the birds from diseases. The enteric organisms like salmonellae and coliforms produce egg borne diseases. Bacteria and many other fungi can even enter the eggshell for further spread of the disease processes. Bacteriological, serological, parasitological, histopathological and animal inoculation tests are done to diagnose the poultry diseases. The duration of the symptoms, the number or size of dead birds, information on ventilation, feeding, watering system, lighting, debeaking, breeding, vaccination, age of birds, weather and history of diseases are important factors for the consideration of pathologists in the diagnosis of poultry diseases. The infection in birds due to retroviruses, picornaviruses, adenoviruses, reoviruses, salmonellae, *E. coli,* mycoplasma and *Aspergillus fumigatus* are transmitted transovarianly (i.e. through the eggs) to the baby chicks.

Impaired body functions, deficiency of vital nutrients, ingestion of toxic substances, injuries, physical stress, infection and parasites etc. cause diseases in birds. A disturbed host parasite relationship culminates in diseases. A mild roundworm infection in birds is not an important disease but severe roundworm infestation may cause emaciation and death in the infected birds. Several organisms present in the environment are not pathogens for birds. Many bacterial or viral diseases are flock diseases that require flock treatment for eradication. Some bacterial or viral diseases are transmitted vertically and horizontally into other birds. Both vertical and horizontal transmissions are noticed in birds infected with reoviruses.

Several factors called immunosuppressents decrease immunity by destroying the lymphoid cells or bursa of Fabricius. The birds having decreased immune response are easy targets to other secondary infections.

The main immunosuppressents are as follows:

1. Viral diseases like infectious bursal disease (Gumboro disease), lymphoid leucosis and retroviral infections
2. Cytotoxic drugs e.g. cortisone, cyclophosphamide and some insecticides
3. Mycotoxins e.g. aflatoxins, ochratoxins and some other fungal toxins
4. Deficiencies of vitamin B, vitamin C, poor diet and starvation etc. produce atrophy in thymus and bursa of Fabricius
5. The stress factors like excessive heat, transportation, deworming, high density of bird, debeaking and excessive ammonia in poultry houses adversely affect the immunity of birds.

Prevalence (incidence) of diseases, age groups and immune status of birds in poultry farm are important factors in working out a vaccination schedule in poultry farm. Poultry vaccines are important tools to boost poultry industry.

Vaccination in birds offers some protection to birds against some other animate infections. Vaccination against M.D.(Marek's disease) in birds reduces incidence of certain other diseases like chronic respiratory disease (CRD), avian leucosis complex (ALC) and coccidiosis in birds. Combined poultry vaccines are used to reduce stress in the poultry flocks. The hatched chicks of vaccinated birds are rich in maternal antibodies (MAB) to offer passive immunity for few days after hatching against viral infections. Knowledge on levels of maternal antibodies in chicks helps in deciding about the age of chickens to be vaccinated. Immunity in some diseases (say, IBD) develops after two weeks of vaccination.

Vaccinated birds are protected against viral infections by interference phenomenon. Vaccination (primary and booster) in chickens of different age groups is carried out to strengthen and maintain resistance (immunity) in flocks.

VIRAL REPLICATION

Knowledge of viral replication in the infected birds helps one to understand infections, disease pathogenesis and effects produced in the body. It also helps in application of the rational steps of disease prevention and control.

The different steps with replication of most DNA viruses include replication of DNA and transcription of RNA from double-stranded DNA. Most DNA viruses replicate in the cell nuclei, using cellular RNA polymerase 2 and other cellular enzymes. But most RNA viruses replicate with in the cytoplasm. Some RNA viruses carry their own RNA polymerase (e.g. virion associated transcriptase) and use to transcribe RNA from the RNA genome whereas genomes of other RNA viruses themselves function as mRNAs for production of virions as exemplified by the picorna viruses and astroviruses. The two general modes of DNA and RNA replications are given in table 1.

Table 1 Viral replication

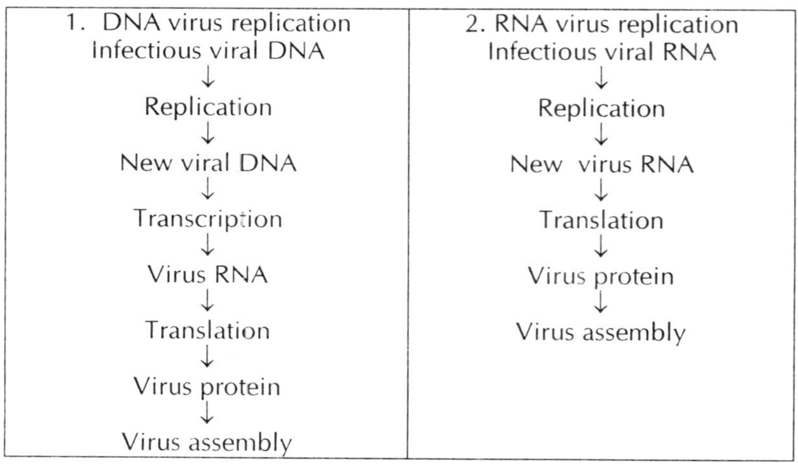

1. DNA virus replication	2. RNA virus replication
Infectious viral DNA	Infectious viral RNA
↓	↓
Replication	Replication
↓	↓
New viral DNA	New virus RNA
↓	↓
Transcription	Translation
↓	↓
Virus RNA	Virus protein
↓	↓
Translation	Virus assembly
↓	
Virus protein	
↓	
Virus assembly	

In retroviruses, the viral genome is integrated into the host cells DNA as a DNA copy (provirus) of viral RNA.

Viral proteins (e.g. capsid proteins) are very toxic to cells and shutdown protein synthesis (i.e. cellular DNA or RNA formation). Birds dying of leucosis show large livers extending up to the vent.

The main effects of the viral infections are as under:

1. Inhibiting host cell DNA, RNA and protein synthesis and creating situation incompatible to life. A virus binds to the cell surface receptors and penetrates into the cells. The enveloped viruses fuse with the plasma membrane. Nonenveloped viruses enter the cells by endocytosis, or pinocytosis. Processes like viral replication, transcription and translation excessively increase viral concentrations in the cells which undergo disintegration or lytic changes.
2. Damaging integrity of cells or plasma membranes promote cell fusion as exemplified by the herpesvirus. Poxvirus acquires membranes probably from the Golgi apparatus and also fuse with the plasma membranes before release of the virions. Some of the pox viruses may be released even without envelopes.
3. Replicating in cells and causing destruction or necrosis of the host cells as shown by cytocidal viruses like herpes or picornaviruses. The body cells infected with unenveloped viruses disintegrate and the viruses are released into the environment.
4. Secondary bacterial infection is seen in the host cells damaged or devitalized by the viruses.
5. Inducing cell proliferation and transformation of normal cells into cancer (e.g. Rous sarcoma virus of the fowl).
6. Cytopathic effects of the viral inclusions on the cells (e.g. damaging effects of intracytoplasmic inclusion bodies in the

pox virus infection) are also noticed in the affected cells. Lysis or necrosis is caused by cytocidal viruses like herpesviruses, picornaviruses and paramyxoviruses. The sites of cellular inclusions in certain poultry diseases are given in table 2.

7. Capsid or neucleocapsid proteins or protein products by the viruses exert very toxic effects on the infected cells. Viruses do not produce toxins as done by certain bacteria.

8. Rounding up, death or lysis of the viral infected cells with the release of the virions and transmission of infection to neighbouring healthy cells by the released virions

9. Haemorrhagic, exudative and necrotic lesions are caused by certain viruses in the affected organs. Haemorrhagic or necrotic lesions are important changes in the digestive tract (e.g. proventriculus, intestine and caecal tonsils etc.) in affected fowls in Ranikhet disease(RD). Exudative lesions may be minimal in some virus diseases. All negative stranded RNA viruses and retroviruses are released through budding. While extruding through the cell membranes, RD viruses acquire envelopes from the cell membranes and cause necrosis of the cells.

Table 2 Sites of inclusions in the cells

Diseases	Sites in cells
1. Infectious laryngotracheitis (ILT)	(i) Intranuclear inclusions in the epithelial cells of the infected laryngeal and tracheal mucosae
2. Avian Pox (AP)	(ii) Eosinophilic cytoplasmic inclusions (Bollinger bodies) in the infected cutaneous ephithelium

10. Accumulation of viral encoded proteins or epidermal growth factors in the infected cells causes excessive mitotic divisions of the dermal or follicular epithelial cells to form nodular

proliferations called pox.

11. Absence of cytopathic effects

No cytoplasmic effects are seen in certain viral infections, but such viruses produce latent or persistent infections. Retroviruses are released from the cells without cellular lysis.

Chronic viral infections arise from persistent infection of virus in the hosts. Infectious carriers arise from chronic infection of viruses.

12. Cell fusion

Some viruses are marked by feature of cell fusion to form synctia. In infected birds by paramyxovirus, herpesvirus or coronavirus, changes in the cell membranes of the infected cells cause fusion of these cells to form synctia. Non-specific changes like acute celluar swelling, increase in permeability of the cell membranes and leakage of the lysosomes in the cellular cytoplasm are also noticed in the cells infected with viruses.

13. Cell lysis

A virus persists in the host cells without its replication in the cells. A herpesvirus infection may be followed by a latent infection. A slow virus infection is a persistent infection with long incubation period as exemplified by maedi or HIV. Specifically sensitized T-lymphocytes and natural killer cells (NK cells) also destroy virus-infected cells.

An immune or cell mediated response causes lysis of the virus-infected cells. Viruses impart new antigens to the surface of infected cells and specifically sensitized T lymphocytes cause destruction of virus-infected cells. Natural killer cells (NK cells) also destroy the virus-infected cells. Spread of virions is limited by death and destruction of the infected cells. Syncytial cell formation is noticed in some viral infections e.g. the infected cells with herpes or paramyxoviruses. Some basic informations regarding main viral diseases in birds are given in table 3.

Table 3 Some important avian viruses and their main pathological signs and lesions in the affected birds

Family	Virus type	Structure of the viral genomes and their important features	Diseases caused	Pathological signs and lesions
(1)	(2)	(3)	(4)	(5)
(A) Poxviridae	Avipox virus	A single molecule of the double stranded (ds)DNA (+/-),replication in the cytoplasm, virions released by budding(enveloped virions) or by cell lysis (non enveloped virions), intracy toplasmic inclusions, transmission by direct contact and presence of virion associated transcriptase	Pox/Fowl pox	1. Discrete nodular proliferative skin lesions on the unfeathered parts in the cutaneous form of the fowl pox. 2. Fibrinonecrotic or diphtheritic necrotic membrane in the mucous membrane of mouth, oesophagus and respiratory tract in diphtheritic form of fowl pox
(B) Retroviridae	Retrovirus—Alpharetro virus (avian type C reterovirus)	Single stranded RNA positive sense virus, replication in nuclei, non-enveloped, DNA step in	Neoplastic diseases of leucosis/sarcoma group	Neoplastic growth is noticed in organs affected with lymphoid leucosis,

(1)	(2)	(3)	(4)	(5)
		replication by reverse transcriptase (viral RNA dependent DNA polymerase). DNA copy (negative sense) of the reterovirus integrating with cellular genome to transform the infected cells into malignant heritable cancer cells e.g. Rous sarcoma of fowls and ALC.DNA copy (provirus)is transcribed to form a RNA		fibroma and fibrosarcoma etc.
(C) Reoviridae	Reovirus	Double stranded RNA virus with negative sense, replication in the cytoplasm, non-enveloped virus transcribed into the positive sense RNA in the cytoplasm with the help of virion associated transcriptase and positive sense RNA acting like templates for replication	Viral arthritis (tenosynovitis)	Lameness in chickens and broilers, immobilised hock joints, straw coloured or blood tinged exudate in the swollen hock joints. Fusion of the tendon sheaths in chronic cases and erosions on the articular cartilage of distal tibiotarsal joints

(1)	(2)	(3)	(4)	(5)
(D) Herpesviridae	Herpes virus (Gallid herpes Virus 2 (i.e.MD Virus)	Linear double stranded (ds) DNA enveloped virions. DNA transcribed in the nuclei of the affected cells with help of DNA dependent RNA polymerase II	Marek's disease	Lymphoproliferative changes, mononuclear infiltration in peripheral nerves, iris, goads, muscle, skin and visceral organs.
(E) Paramyxoviridae	Paramyxovirus ype(PMV I)	Linear single stranded RNA, negative sense, presence of virion associated transcriptase (RNA dependent RNA polymerase), replication In cytoplasm and transcription of viral RNA into mRNA. In the replication mode, transcription produces a full length positive sense mRNA which acts like a template for the synthesis of new negative sense viral RNA and the	Ranikhet disease (Newcastle disease)	1.Gasping, mouth breathing, greenish diarrhoea and fluid in the crop of infected birds 2. Presence of nervous and paralytic symptoms 3. Haemorrhages at the oesophagus/ proventriculus and proventriculus/gizzard junctions and such haemorrhages or petechiae in the small

(1)	(2)	(3)	(4)	(5)
		enzyme polymerase (RNA dependent RNA polymerase) acts like a replicase and the transcription involves the role of virion associated transcriptase		intestines and caecal tonsils are virtually pathogonomonic lesions of Ranikhet disease
(F) Picornaviridae	1. Picornavirus 2. Three types of duck hepatitis virus (1) Duck hepatitis virus type 1 (a picornavirus) (2) Duck hepatitis virus 2 (an astrovirus) (3) Duck hepatitis virus 3 (a picornavirus—an unrelated type to DHV type 1)	A linear single stranded RNA positive sense non enveloped virus, replication in cytoplasm and direct transcription. The genomic RNAs or RNA viruses of positive sense act as messenger RNA	1. Avian encephalomyelitis (epidemic tremor) 2. Duck hepatitis	1. Ataxia, quick tremors or a vibratory movement of the head and neck, coma and death in the sick birds 2. White streaks in the muscularis of ventriculus and non-purulent encephalomyelitis marked by perivascular cuffing, ne-uronal degeneration and gliosis.

(1)	(2)	(3)	(4)	(5)
(G) Birinaviridae	Avibirna virus	Double stranded RNA genome, replication in cytoplasm, non-enveloped, viral replication similar to that of Reovirus	Infectious bursal disease. (IBD) Young chickens severally affected	1.Immunosuppression in the sick birds 2. Destruction of lymphoid structures like spleen and bursa of Fabricius 3. Oedema, hyperaemic and haemorrhagic changes in the cloacal bursa of the dead birds are pathognomonic lesions in IBD 4. Atrophy of bursa at later stages
(H) Coronaviridae	Coronavirus	Single stranded RNA virus, positive sense, replication in cytopolasm and enveloped virions	Infectious bronchitis Chickens affected.	1. Tracheal rales, sneezing, coughing, nasal discharge in young chickens. Decreased egg production in layers

(1)	(2)	(3)	(4)	(5)
				2. Catarrhal or caseous exudate in the trachea, nasal passages and sinuses. 3. Infiltration of heterophils and lymphocytes in the tracheal mucosa.
(l) Orthomyxovirid ae	Orthomyxovirus Influenza type 'A'	Linear segmented single stranded RNA, negative sense and presence of transcriptase in the RNA virions.	Avian influenza, chickens and turkeys affected and an important zoonosis	1. Cough, sneezing, rales, emaciation and decreased feed consumption in the sick birds 2. Lacrimation, huddling, oedema in unfeathered parts 3. Mortality and morbidity up to 100% 4. Degenerative or nec-rotic changes in the liver and kidneys and focal necrosis in the brain and skeletal musles

(1)	(2)	(3)	(4)	(5)
				5. Presence of perivascular lymphoid cuffing in organs like heart and lungs etc.
(J) Herpesviridae	Galid herpes virus I	A DNA virus, formation of intranuclear inclusions in the epithelial cells of trachea	Laryngotracheitis in chickens of all ages	1. Head shaking, gasping and dyspnoea in sick birds.
(K) Astroviridae	Astrovirus (Duck hepatitis virus 2)	A single molecule of linear single stranded RNA virus, positive sense, replication in cytoplsam, viral genome functioning directly as mRNA. In other words, RNA virus binds directly to ribosomes and is then translated.	Duck heptatitis The other causative viruses are DHV1 and DHV3	1.Spasmodic contraction of both legs, partially closed eyes, polydypsia, loose droppings, excessive urates excretion and falling or dropping on their sides. 2. Enlarged livers with haemorrhages, massive necrosis of hepatocytes, regenerative changes in the liver cells and bile duct hyperplasia

(1)	(2)	(3)	(4)	(5)
(L) Adenoviridae	Aviadenovirus	A single molecule of linear double stranded (ds) DNA (+/-), replication in the nuclei and transcription leads to production of monocistronic mRNAs.	Egg drop syndrome	Fall in egg production, inflammatory changes in the pouch shell gland and thin soft shelled eggs with loss of colour or pigmentation in the eggs

Bacterial infections

Salmonellosis, a serious hazard to growing poultry industry in a country, is an egg-borne disease. Humans are prone to danger of transovarian transmission of salmonellosis. Endotoxins released by salmonellae greatly damage the birds. Fowl typhoid and pullorum disease cause septicaemic infections in poultry. Paratyphoid infection in birds caused by a very common *Salmonella* like *Salmonella enteritidis* is a toxaemic disease by endotoxins associated with this *Salmonella* spp. There is also direct ovarian transmission of paratyphoid (PT) infection in the birds. *E. coli* infection causes septicaemia in birds. Granulomatous lesions due to *E. coli* are noticed in the guts of birds infected with Hjärre's disease. Fowl cholera is a haemorrhagic septicaemic disease in the fowls with high mortality. *Pasteurella multocida* produces powerful endotoxins. *Mycobacterium tuberculosis avium* causes tuberculosis in birds.

Several types of *M. avium* have been isolated from humans. However, man is resistant to *M. avium* infection. Avian tuberculosis is a chronic and progressive disease in natural hosts.

Clostridium type C excretes a type C toxin that causes botulism in birds. Avian botulism (limberneck in birds) is marked by flaccid paralysis of legs, wings, neck and eyelids. Wings drop due to paralysis. The term limberneck especially refers to paralysis of neck. Free type C toxin binds to the cell membrane, translocates and reacts interacellularly to block release of acetylacholine from synaptic vesicles. The cholinergic nerve endings are motor end plates and as such, inhibition of the release of acetylcholine leads to paralysis of muscles.

Effects of bacterial infection depend upon the ability of the bacteria to cause disease (i.e. virulence). Only organisms causing diseases are called pathogens. On entering the tissues, bacteria produce enzymes like hyaluronidase, collagenase and elastase, which split connective tissuses, structure molecules, hyaluronic acid, collagen and elastin respectively. The extra cellular matrix opens up and the bacteria are allowed to move and propagate between the cells. Some other bacteria secrete enzymes to destroy fibrin.

Cells nutrients, oxygen and proteins etc. are consumed by bacteria. As a result of this, the nearby cells die of starvation. Bacteria penetrate into the cell and multiply intracellularly. Invading bacteria release toxins during intercellular growth. The secreted toxic materials by bacteria are called exotoxins (proteins in nature). *Clostridium tetani* produces a toxin called tetanospasmin, which is activated by proteolytic enzymes in the tissues. The tetanospasmin travels from the site of bacterial growth along the nerves to the spines. The inhibitory neurons are suppressed with excessive activity of the nerves to end in serve muscular contraction (tetanic spasms). Later, paralysis of the muscles or organs is noticed in the animal patients.

Endotoxins have components like polysaccharides, lipids and proteins etc. in the cells of certain bacteria (e.g. gram negative bacteria), anthrax bacilli and mycobacteria of avian type etc. Following disintegration of bacterial bodies, endotoxins are released. The toxic properties of the endotoxins depend on lipids. A fraction (a specific fraction), which causes release of cellular proteins, is called cytokine. The liberated cytokines are responsible for fever, malaise, hypertension and shock etc.in the affected animals. Such condition in animal patients is called septic shock.

Genetic diseases

Genetic diseases are diseases caused by defective genes. The defective genes are formed due to X-radiation and certain chemical agents. Genetic abnormalities result in defective amino acid metabolism, defective lipid metabolism, defective purine metabolism and so on. Some hereditary diseases may be sexlinked and are expressed by only one sex. The crooked neck syndrome in brown leghorns is attributed to a single recessive gene and resembles crooked neck syndrome of turkeys, which is an osteodystrophy of the cervical vertebrae.

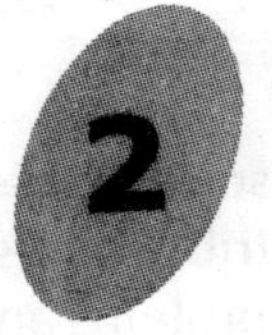

Ranikhet Disease (Newcastle Disease)

It is an acute viral contagious disease of fowls which are the chiefly affected birds with the first report of them in Jawa in 1926. Turkeys are also susceptible to it. Ducks, pigeons and geese may also be attacked by it. Infection spreads through contaminated food or water with infective excretions and faeces etc. Ranikhet disease virus is considered as paramyxovirus type-1 (PMV-1) infection of paramyxoviridae group of the enveloped RNA viruses.

The five pathotypes of RDV are given in **Table 4:**

Incubation period varies from 5 to 7 days. The mortality may go up to 100%. The virus produces conjunctivitis and lymphadenitis in man. Birds of all ages are susceptible to Ranikhet disease. The disease spreads by direct or indirect contact. The virus of Ranikhet disease may survive in the infected premises for 2 to 3 weeks. Viscerotropic (velogenic) NDV causes Doyle's form of NDV marked by haemorrhagic or necrotic lesions in the intestinal tract. Neurotropic velogenic NDV produces nervous and respiratory symptoms or lesions in poultry. Indian deshi birds are not only resistant to RDV but also act like carriers.

Viral replication

RDV (Ranikhet disease virus) is a single stranded virus having negative sense which is first attached to cell receptors of the avain host. Fusion of the viral and cell membranes is followed by entry of the nucleocapsid into the cells. Cellular cytoplasm is the site of intracellular viral replication. RD virus which has negative sense RNA genome cannot act as a messenger RNA and it so uses RNA virion associated RNA directed RNA polymerase (virion transcriptase) to produce complementary transcripts of positive sense which act as mRNAs utilising the cellular mechanism (ribosomes) for protein synthesis and RNA is translated into proteins and viral genomes. The viral proteins synthesised in the intected cells are transferred to the cell membranes. Finally, viral particles are budded from the cell surfaces as enveloped viruses.

The NDV first replicates in the mucosal epithelium of the upper respiratory and intestinal tracts. It is soon followed by spread of the virus via the blood to the spleen and bone marrow, producing thus the state of viraemia. This leads to infection of other organs like lungs and central nervous system. Damage to the respiratory centre in the brain is produced. As a result, respiratory distress and dyspnoea are seen in the sick birds. Petechiae or ecchymotic haemorrhages are noticed in many organs like pharynx, trachea, and oesophagus, proventriculus and intestine etc. Lymphatic tissue and intestinal mucosae reveal necrotic changes. Virus strains of NDV (like those of high, intermediate and low virulence) are represented by terms like velogenic (viscerotropic), mesogenic and lentogenic types. Haemorrhages produced by viscerotropic Asiatic virus at the proventriculus/oesophagus and proventriculus/gizzard junctions along with the haemorrhages in the posterior half of duodenum, jejunum, ileum and caecal tonsils are virtually pathognomonic for velogenic strains of RDV in Asiatic countries like India. Encephalomyelitis marked by neuronal necrosis, perivascular cuffing and interstitial inflamatory infiltrations are seen in central nervous system of the affected birds.

Signs

Staggering, torticollis, diarrhoea, opisthotonus and nervous symtoms can be present in the birds. Gasping inhalations through half opened beak, thick mucous discharge and a watery yellowish or greenish diarrhoea with an obnoxious odour are some of the main signs of this disease. The Newcastle disease is a respiratory disease in the United States. But in India, viscerotropic lesions like those in the alimentary tract are very remarkable changes. When respiratory symptoms with tracheitis and haemorrhages

Table 4

Forms of paramyxovirus infections (diseases)	Causes (pathotypes of viruses)	Main features
1. Doyle's or Asiatic form Viscerotropic Velogenic Newcastle disease (VVND)	NDV strains of high virulence (VVND pathotype)	1. Acute lethal infection marked by 100% i.e. high mortality in the Asiatic type. 2. Gasping, mouth breathing, torticollis and paralysis. 3. Haemorrhages, especially in the heart, proventriculus, gizzard, intestine, ovaries and brain. Tracheitis with haemorrhages and haemmorhages and necrotic lesions in the digestive tract (particularly in the duodenum, ileum and caecal tonsils). Green diarrhoea is frequently seen in sick birds.
2. Beach's form Neurotropic Velogenic Newcastle disease (NVND)	NVND pathotype	1. Acute lethal infection in chicks of all age groups with 100% morbidity i.e. mortality is lower in the disease form of American type. 2. Respiratory and nervous symptoms arising from pneumoencephalitis are noticed. 3.Hyperaemic and oedematous parabronchi and haemorhages in the alveolar spaces. 4. Fall in egg production and remarkable abscence of diarrhoea in sick birds

Forms of paramyxovirus infections (diseases)	Causes (pathotypes of viruses)	Main features
3. Beaudette's form a less pathogenic form of NVND	*Mesogenic pathotype* and viral strains of intermediate virulence	1. A repiratory form of disease usually affecting the young chicks. 2. Marked by decrease in egg production
4. Hitchner's form	Lentogenic pathotype i.e. strain of low virulence	1. Inapparent respiratory viral infection. 2. Viral types used as vaccines 3. Adult birds usually not affected
5. Asymptomatic enteric form	Lentogenic pathotype or viral strain of low virulence	1. Marked by no obvious disease in poultry 2. Gut infections may be caused by lentogenic viruses.

are prominent in the birds, tracheal rales and crackling sounds can be heard. The birds are depressed, their eyes are closed and are unable to use one or both legs. Nervous or paralytic symptoms may be found in the affected birds.

Pathology

Presence of haemorrhages on the gizzard, pericardial sac and mucosae of the proventriculus is a very important set of lesions which aid in its diagnosis. The crop can be found distended with greyish brown sour-smelling fluid. There is presence of haemorrhagic necrotic enteritis as seen in duodenum, jejunum and ileum. Petechiae and necrotic changes are also found in the caecal tonsils. The virus of RD can be found in the body fluid, internal organs and excretion etc. In Doyle's form of RD, haemorrhagic and necrotic lesions are found in the intestinal wall but in other form of ND or RD, the primary lesions are found in the respiratory tract. Thickening of airsacs or pnemonia can be noticed in the latter kind of infected birds. Haemorrhages or inflammatory changes are noticed in some organs. Airsacs are also inflamed and congested. Tracheal mucosae may show haemorrhages.

Diagnosis

It is based on the symptoms, lesions (for example, characteristic petechiae on the mucous membrane of proventriculus and caecal tonsils), the haemagglutination inhibition test and ELISA etc.

TREATMENT/CONTROL

Treatment is not very beneficial because of very high mortality up to 100% in the birds affected with Ranikhet disease virus (PMV-1). Only control measures are useful. These are as follows :

(i) The birds are to be given active immunity to control themselves against Ranikhet disease.

(ii) The vaccines (F, R2B and LaSota) are used for this purpose (Table 5). LaSota or F strain is used for intranasal or intraocular vaccination in day-old chicks and revaccination is taken up at 4 weeks to 8 weeks of age by intramuscular route with Mukteshwar R2B vaccine. The birds can react severely with mortality, lameness and paralysis. The immunity given to birds lasts about a year. The healthy birds can be given Vimeral syrup as antistress factor after vaccination and during outbreaks

Precautions

(1) Newcastle disease (F) vaccine (living) is generally administered to the chicks of 5 to 6 days of age.

(2) Marek's disease vaccine is administered to day-old chicks.

(3) NDF is repeated within 8-10 days before administration of R2B vaccine. It is the interference phenomenon which protects the vaccinated birds during a viral outbreak in a flock.

(4) Ranikhet (R2B) vaccine is given to birds at 5 to 6 weeks of age by intramuscular route.

(5) R2B vaccine is repeated at 10th to 14th day after NDF vaccination. Broilers can be given the vaccine at 3-4 weeks of age.

(6) NDV killed vaccine is given to broilers at any age by intramuscular or subcutanous route. NDV killed vaccine boosts up immunity in layers which are administered at 16 to 20 weeks of age.

(7) Combined Newcastle disease (La Sota) and intectious bronchitis (Ma5 type) vaccine can be used to vaccinate the chickens at 3-4 weeks of age by intramuscular route. Layers can also be administered at 15-16 weeks of age and also at 40 to 42 weeks in drinking water.

(8) Inactivated RDV, IB and IBD vaccine is given to breeders by intramuscular or subcutaneous route at 2-4 weeks before egg laying. The newly-hatched chicks from the eggs of such

Table 5 Vaccination programme as a guide line for immunity against some poultry diseases

Age	Diseases	Vaccines	Route	Remarks
(1)	(2)	(3)	(4)	(5)
Day 1	Marek's disease	Marek's disease vaccine	Subcutaneous in the neck region	Protection against MD within 7 days postvaccination
Day 0-3	Infectious bursal disease (IBD)	IBD (Gumboro) mild vaccine/IBD Lukert (mild strain) vaccine	Intraocular, one drop in each eye	Level of maternal antibodies may be checked.
Day 4-7	ND/ND+IB (infectious bronchitis)	NDVF vaccine/La Sota strain/Clone 30 (Intervet) plus Ma5 (Massachusetts strain 5) i.e. Ma5+Clone 30	Intranasal or intraocular one drop in each nostril	Immunity against ND up to 4 months of age by the 1st Lasota vaccination
Day 14	IBD	Gumboro vaccine Nobilis, strain D78/Gumboro vaccine Nobilis 228E	Intraocular, one drop in each eye or drinking water	Layers and broilers from day 14 to 21
Day 21	ND	NDV vaccine F strain/La Sota strain/Clone 30 (Intervet)	Intraocular or drinking water	
Day 28	IBD	IBD intermediate/ Gumboro vaccine 228 E (Georgia strain)	Intraocular or drinking water	

(1)	(2)	(3)	(4)	(5)
Week 6-8	ND (Newcastle disease)	NDV-R2B (Mukteswar) strain vaccine	Subcutaneous or intramuscular	
Week 8	Fowl pox	Fowlpox vaccine	Wing web method (two pricks)	Life-long immunity
Week 16	ND+IBD+IB	Combined inactivated vaccine against infectious bursal disease, Newcastle disease and infectious bronchitis	Subcutaneous/ intramuscular	
Week 8-16 Avian Encephalomy elitis	Avian encephalo-myelitis	A.E. vaccine Nobilis	Drinking water	Birds also protected against egg drop syndrome and full immunity established within 2 to 3 weeks after vaccination.

vaccinated birds are rich in maternal antibodies. In case of immunosuppression due to IBD infection, chickens can be given inactivated ND, IB and IBD vaccines between 14 and 21 days. While administering Gumbro vaccine, the level of maternal antibodies is a deciding factor about the age of chickens chosen for vaccination against Gumboro disease.

(9) Instructions given by manufacturers for a particular vaccine are carefully read before use.

(10) Inactivated vaccines are preferred to be administered between 16 and 20 weeks of age.

(11) Thigh and breast muscles are chosen for intramuscular injection. Leg or the back of the neck is a good site for subcutaneous injection.

(12) Only healthy birds need to be vaccinated.

(13) Allow the inactivated vaccine to reach the temperature of 5-25°C before use.

(14) Breeders and layers around 16 to 20 weeks of age are preferred for administration of inactivated vaccines.

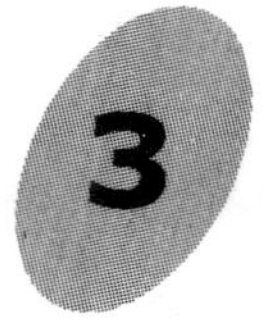

Infectious Bursal Disease (Gumboro Disease)

This disease is a contagious RNA viral disease (a birnavirus infection of the Birnaviridae family) in chickens with the greatest incidence in chickens of 3-6 weeks of age. The clinical signs of the disease can be seen in the birds for 5-7 days after infection of the flock and the mortality rate may rise up to 20-30%. This virus shows a severe reaction in the whiteleg horns and has got a high specificity for the bursa of Fabricius. Water, feed and droppings from the infected stock remain very infectious for 52 days. The meal worms *Alphitobius diaperinus* after an outbreak has been found to be infectious for susceptible birds and can spread the infection to healthy birds. It has a short incubation period of about 2 days.

Signs

There is a tendency in the infected birds to pick at their own vent. The infected birds show soiled vent feathers, whitish or watery diarrhoea, anorexia, depression, ruffled feathers, marked trembling and prostration etc. The birds suffer from dehydration and subnormal temperature in the terminal stages of the disease. The morbidity in the birds may reach 100% and the ruffled feathers and droopy appearance are very important signs of the disease. The birds show mortality from 3rd day after infection which falls in a period of 5-7 days. The initial outbreaks of this disease are quite acute ones. Chickens show age predisposition to it. Immunosuppression is noticed in the infected birds. Increased susceptibility to diseases like coccidiosis, Ranikhet disease, MD, fowl cholera and salmonellosis etc. are noticed in the birds recovered from infectious bursal disease.

PATHOLOGY

Gross changes

The main changes are :

1. Dehydrated and darkened discolouration of the pectoral muscles
2. Frequent haemorrhages in the thigh and pectoral muscles
3. Increased mucus in the intestine. Haemorrhages are noticed at the juncture of the proventriculus and gizzard
4. Extreme damage to the kidneys. These are enlarged and their tubules are distended with accumulated urates.
5. The spleen may be enlarged with small grey foci.
6. After viral infection, the bursa shows increase in size from 3rd day due to oedema and hyperaemia and may be double the size of normal bursa on the 4th day. Later, it shows decrease in size and by 5th day, it returns to normal size. Bursa of Fabricius has a gelatinous yellowish exudate over the serosal surface on the 2nd or 3rd day postinfection. The internal striations of the bursa are prominent and have cream coloured appearance. When atrophy of the bursa sets in, it becomes grey in colour. The bursa in the diseased birds has necrotic foci and petechial or ecchymotic haemorrhages on the mucosal surface. Haemorrhages can be seen in patches of different sizes in the skin or abdominal regions of the body. B-lymphocytes within the bursa are mostly destroyed. Oedema and haemorrhage in bursa are typical changes in acute experimental IBD at 3-4 days postinfection of IBD virus.

Microscopic changes

The bursal lesions are even seen from the 1st day of infection i.e. 1st day post infection. Degeneration and necrosis of lymphocytes are seen in the medullary areas. Later, heterophils, pyknotic debris and hyperplastic reticuloendothelial cells are also seen. Haemorrhages are often present. Severe oedema, hyperaemia and marked accumulation of lymphocytes are seen in the bursa of the infected birds. Bursal epithelial cells also proliferate to form cells of glandular structures containing globules of mucin. Lymphoid cells forming discrete follicles with little interfollicular tissue are seen in the sections of bursa stained by H & E method. Interfollicular oedema mixed with phagocytes is also seen. Degenerative changes are seen in the follicles. Only ghosts of the follicles can be seen with phagocytic role of heterophils. Proliferation of the reticuloendothelial cells around the adenoid sheath arteries of the spleen and lymphoid necrosis can be seen in this organ. There is presence of large casts of homogenous material infiltrated by hetrophils in the kidneys. The livers may show slight perivascular infiltration of lymphocytes. Lymphocidal effect is the marked lesion in the bursa, spleen, thymus and tonsils.

Diagnosis

It is based on the following :

1. Signs and lesions of the disease
2. The gross enlargement and pink colouration of the bursa of Fabricius is quite characteristic and **pathognomonic**.
3. Virus neutralisation test
4. The ELISA test to detect IBDV antibodies. This test confirms the IBDV infection in a very short period.
5. The group antigen of the IBDV can also be detected by gel diffusion and immunofluoresence.

TREATMENT/MANAGEMENT

No specific treatment is available. Antistress drugs like both B-complex or vimeral syrup can be orally given to birds. The chicks after hatching from the eggs have natural maternal antibodies to be protected against (IBDV) for a period of one week.

Vaccination can only be reliable to control the disease and for this, live attenuated freeze dried vaccine is available (Table 5). The birds between the age group of 0-5 days can be vaccinated with D 78 (Intervet). Killed vaccine can be used by oral or intraocular route.Since Gumboro disease is caused by a RNA virus which destroys the immune system of body like AIDS virus in humans. levamisole can be used as an immunomodulator or potentiator. Vitamin A, E, and C can also be given.

Infectious bursal disease vaccine or IBD inactivated vaccine can be given to the chickens by subcutatneous (neck region) or intramuscular (thigh or pectoral muscles) route.

A combined vaccine against IB, Gumboro disease and NCD is also available for use in chickens. This vaccine saves the birds from the stress of a second vaccination.

Marek's Disease (MD)

It is a lymphoproliferative disease of chickens caused by a virus (i.e. a herpes virus). There is a characteristic mononuclear infiltration of peripheral nerves but such infiltration can also occur in the gonads, iris, various viscera, muscle and skin etc. There is a gross enlargement of the peripheral nerves due to mononuclear infiltration which also causes paralysis in the birds. Mononuclear infiltration of the iris causes depigmentation or greyish opacity and birds develop blindness or grey eyes or ocular lymphomatosis. Leucotic lesions are produced in visceral organs (eg. proventriculus) or even skin. Marek's disease in chickens occurs in India and several other countries i.e. the world over. 25 to 30 percent of the affected birds may die in the outbreak of MD. The virus of this disease has been isolated from the feather follicle epithelium. The core of this herpes virus has been found to contain DNA and the virus multiplies in the nucleus. Apart from causing degenerative changes in the lymphoid tumour cells, tumours in the visceral organs, skin and muscle are also formed by the virus. The virus of this disease infects turkeys and pheasants etc. The disease can spread to other birds from the infected ones by direct or indirect contact or by air-borne particles of the faeces or droppings etc. The infected birds which survive attack of MD can act as carriers of this infection. Egg transmission of this disease is quite insignificant. Outbreaks of MD are found in the birds as young as 3-4 weeks but serious outbreaks are found after the 8th or 9th week of age. In short, pullets and cockrels are susceptible from 4 to 12 months of age and birds over 12 months of age are resistant. The incubation period may vary from 3 to 4 weeks in some cases and may be many months in others. The MD virus reaches infectious stage in the skin epithelium and is shed along with the dander and feathers in the environment. The virus survives in the litter dust and poultry house for about 4-8 months in shaded places.

Signs

The chief signs are :

1. Weakness and paralysis of one or more of the extremities
2. Drooping of the wings
3. Head may be held low, torticollis may be present due to involvement of cervical nerves and paralysis or dilation of the crop or gasping owing to vagal paralysis is noticed in the sick birds.
4. Incoordination of movements in the affected birds
5. One leg may be streched forward whereas the other may be stretched backward. Lameness or paralysis of one or both legs or wings is noticed in birds around 3 months or more in age in classical MD infections.
6. Severe depression
7. Presence of dehydration, emaciation and coma
8. Blindness due to involvement of the iris
9. Depigmentation or bluish grey opacity of the eyes with irregular appearance of pupil
10. Weight loss, paleness, anorexia and diarrhoea may be present.
11. Morbidity and mortality are nearly equal. Females are more susceptible than males in a flock. It is inavariably fatal in few weeks and recovery from the disease is rare.

PATHOLOGY

Gross changes

These are as follows:

(1) Enlargement of the sciatic nerves and brachial plexus. The

coeliac plexus is involved in 78% of the sick birds. There is loss of striations with grey or yellow discolouration of the peripheral nerves. These nerves may also be oedematous in appearance. The enlargement of the sciatic nerve or brachial plexus is often unilateral.

(2) Lympoid tumors of greyish soft discolouration are present in the gonad (especially the ovary). Such lesions are also found in the lungs, heart, mesentery, proventriculus, intestine, iris, skelatal muscle and skin etc. Leucotic tumours in these organs are quite indistinguishable from those caused by lymphoid leucosis virus in such organs. Tumour-like growths are found in the lungs. The liver may be enlarged or may have granular appearance due to lymphoid hyperplasia in its substance. Leucotic tumours may be found in the ovaries which may have cauliflower-like appearance. The proventriculus may be thickened. Diffuse infiltration or nodular neoplastic formation can be present the in heart. Diffuse whitish nodules or swollen feather follicles can also be found in the skin. Tumours are rarely formed in the bursa of Fabricius in the MD viral infection.

Microscopic appearance

The main changes are :

1. Heavy infiltration of the mononuclear cells in the peripheral nerve fibres, oedema, myelin degeneration and Schwann cell proliferation may be present. A mixture of cells like small and medium lymphocytes, plasma cells and lymphoblasts and macropohages may be found in the thickened nerves.

2. Presence of Marek's disease cells which are basophilic, pyroninophilic cells having vacuolated cytoplasm and a nucleus with little or no details.

The main changes in the nerves of the chickens affected with Marek's disease are as follows :

(i) Infiltration of inflammatory cells at first occurs perivascularly in the nerves and replacement of the nerves or tissues by massive increase of cells which include lymphocytes, plasma cells and some lymphoblasts. There may be little oedema in such affected nerves. Such lesions are called type-1 lesions.

(ii) The type-2 lesions in the nerves are in the form of oedema and few infiltrative cells (mostly plasma cells). There may be occasional fibrosis.

(iii) In type-3 lesions, there is a massive infiltration of neoplastic cells (lymphoblastic cells) in the nerves which frequently show mitotic figures. In short, the lesions in the Marek's disease consist of both inflammatory and degenerative reactions (i.e. infiltration of plasma cells, oedema and fibrosis etc.) as well as the neoplastic cellular infiltrative changes in the affected nerves. In experimental cases of MD in chickens, the lesions consist of proliferating lymphoid cells, demylination and Schwann cell proliferation. Oedema and infiltration of plasma cells and small lymphocytes are also noticed. Perivascular cuffs with densely-staining lymphocytes are seen in the brain. In the MD-affected birds, lymphoid cells or mononuclear infiltration is seen in the iris which may be grey leading to blindness.

Lymphomatotic lesions in the visceral organs are mostly proliferative in nature and consist of lymphocytes and lymphoblasts, Marek's disease cell and some activated reticulum cells. The plasma cells in such lesions are rarely seen. In the skin, the lesions of MD are mostly of inflammatory nature. Massive accumulation of mononuclear cells around the feather follicles, perivascular aggregates of proliferating cells and some presence of plasma cells and histiocytes are seen in the dermis of the infected birds.

Diagnosis

It is based on the following:

1. Symptoms and lesions in the diseased birds

2. Isolation and identification of the MD virus
3. Agar gel difussion test for serological evidence of MD

   The indirect fluorescent antibody and indirect haemagglutination test can also be done to diagnose MD cases.
4. ELISA (Enzyme-linked immunosorbent assay) test

TREATMENT/CONTROL

There is no specific treatment with recovery in sick birds. After this disease has been confirmed in a flock, it is better to do vaccination only in those chickens which are day-old ones (table 5). HVT (Fc-126 strain) live attenuated freeze dried vaccine can be used immediately after hatching from the eggs. The vaccinated chicks are reared in isolation for at least 7 days.

Vaccination of chicks can be done within first three weeks by subcutaneous route. In short, it can be stated that vaccination in day-old chicks and chicks within 1st three weeks can save them from high mortality. Insecticides are used to kill the beetles (*Alphitobius diaperinus*) which can carry the virus for several weeks.

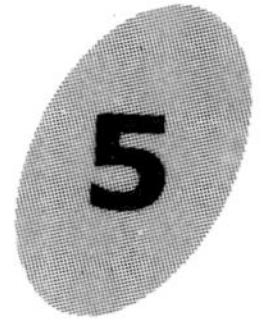

Leucosis/Sarcoma

The leucosis/sarcoma viruses (ALSV of the family Retroviridae) produce different kinds of leucoses which are as follows :

(1) Lymphoid leucosis (big liver disease)

(2) Erythroblastosis (erythroleucosis)

(3) Myeloblastosis (myeloid leucosis)

(4) Myelocytomatosis (a leukaemic myeloid leucosis)

(5) Endothelioma (an endothelial tumour)

(6) Nephroblastoma (embroyonal nephroma)

(7) Hepato-carcinoma (an epithelial tissue tumour)

(8) Fibrosarcoma and fibroma (a connective tissue tumour)

(9) Oesteopetrosis (Thick leg disease)

The retroviruses of this group have common characteristics and a common group specific complement fixing antigen. The myeloblastosis virus has a RNA composition. Rous sarcoma virus and other sarcoma viruses cause neoplastic formation on inoculation in the wing by subcutaneous route. The sarcoma group of viruses produces solid turmours of connective tissue. Rous sarcoma virus produces sarcomas at the site of inoculation. All the viruses (avian types retroviuses)of this group produce tumours in chickens. The viruses are transmitted vertically from parents to offsprings or horizontally from birds to birds (i.e. among the incontact birds). These are shed into egg allbumin to pass finally into the egg chick embryo with perpetuation of the virus infection in the affected flocks.

The lymphoid leucosis occurs at any time after 14 weeks of age with the highest incidence at about sexual maturity. The retroviruses of the leucosis/sarcoma group have been placed in a subgroup of avian type oncoviruses of the family Retroviridae and the differences in leucoses are given in Table 6.

Table 6. The main distinguishing signs and lesions of some tumours produced by the viruses (lecucosis\sarcoma).

Signs and Lesions	Types of Leucoses caused by ALSV Group of Virsues
1. Pale, shrivelled and cyanotic comb, presence of inapptence, emaciation and weakness. Abdomen often enlarged. Feathers spotted with urates and bile. Enlargement of liver, bursa of Fabricius and kidneys felt on palpation. Visible tumours in the liver, spleen and bursa of Fabricius. Tumours are also found in the kidneys, lungs, heart, gonad, bonemarrow and mesentery. The tumours may be miliary or diffuse, soft, smooth and glistening.The tumour cells prolfiferate, displace and compress the cells of the affected organs. Tumours represent aggregate of lymphoid cells. Such lesions are commonly seen in the field cases after 14 weeks of age. The cellular elements of the blood show no significant changes. The lymphoblasts are large in size and have large eccentric nuclei with spongy chromatin and basophilic cytoplasm. These mainly infiltrate extravascularly.	Lymphoid leucosis
2. Presence of erythroblasts in circulation. Marked anaemia. The	Erythroblastosis

birds are lethargy and have general weakness and combs may be pale, cyanotic or almost white. Presence of weakness, anaemia, emaciation and haemorrhages from feather follicles, patechial haemorrhages in the muscles, subcutis and viscera etc. Thrombosis, infarction or ruputure of the liver. Oedema of the lungs, hydropericardium, ascites and fibrinous clot on the surface of the liver. Proliferative changes cause enlargement of the liver and spleen and these organs may be cherry red or dark mahogany colour with soft consistency. The organs are of friable nature. The bone marrow is soft, watery, dark blood red or cherry red and hyperplastic changes are present in it. In anaemic form, the bone marrow is pale or a jelly like substance and spleen may be atrophied. Microscopically, the bone marrow shows blood sinusoids filled with proliferating erythroblasts (failing to mature). Dilatation of the sinusoids is noticed in the liver, spleen and bone marrow. The primary cells involved are erythroblasts in this neoplasm. Erythroblasts are seen in the blood smear.

3.	Paleness of the comb. Lethargy is seen in the birds which are anaemic. Inappetance, emaciation, diarrhoea and dehydration present.	Myeloblastosis

	Description	Diagnosis
	Haemorrhages from feather follicles. Parenchymatous organs may be enlarged or firm. Bone marrow is firm or reddish grey in colour. Liver, spleen and kidneys have greyish infiltrations and mottled appearance. Microscopically, there is presence of massive intravascular and extravascular accumulations of myeloblasts. Infiltrations of such cells are seen in the liver lobules. This differs from erythroblastosis in which there is uniform accumulation of erythroblasts intravascularly. In the bone marrow, the myeloblastic activity is seen in the extrasinusoidal areas. Myeloblastic myeloblasts (comprising 75% of all the cells) are found in the peripheral blood.	
4.	Clinical signs as seen in erythroblastosis are present. Tumours found on the surface of the bones in association with periosteum and nearby cartilage at the costochondral junctions of the bone. These tumours are dull and yellowish white in colour. Microscopically, the tumours consist of masses of uniform myelocytes with very little stroma. The cytoplasm of the myelocytes has acidophilic granules and the nuclei of the cells are vesicular with distinct nucleoli.	Myelocytomatosis
5.	Blood blisters in the skin or on the surface of the visceral organs.	Haemangioma

	Profuse haemorrhages in the skin. The feathers near the tumour are stained with blood. The birds are pale and die of exsanguination. Microscopically, there are cavernoses i.e. distended blood spaces with thin walls composed of endothelial cells.	
6.	Presence of emaciation or debility. Paralysis due to pressure of the tumour on the sciatic nerve. Presence of pinkish grey nodules in the kidneys. These yellowish grey lobulated masses may replace renal parenchyma.The tumours may be pendunculated and connected to kidneys by stalks. Microscopoically, enlarged tubules with invaginated epithelium and well formed glomeruli are found. Irregular masses of distorted tubules are also found. Cystic tubules may be found.	Nephroblastoma
7.	Uniform or irregular thickenings of the diphyseal or metaphyseal regions can be felt by palpation. There is bone-like appearance of the shanks. The affected birds limp or walk with the stilted gait. There is also stunted growth. The periosteum is thickened and the abnormal bones of the limbs are spongy. Basophilic osteoblasts are increased in size and number in the periosteum. Shanks have boot-like appearance. Seen in birds (aged 8-12 weeks).	Osteopetrosis

8.	Benign or malignant tumours are noticed. There is rapid infiltration and metastasis in the malignant tumours. Rous sarcoma virus affects the fibroblastic cells and produce connective tissue tumours. Viruses isolated from lymphoid leucosis also produce fibrosarcomas or myxosarcomas etc. Tumours ulcerate and show metastasis, Fibromas, myxomas and sarcomas are found in the muscles or in the integument. Tumours are also found in bones or cartilage. Fibromas and fibrosarcomas are attached as firm lumps to the skin and seen in the subcutaneous region. The fibromas consist of mature fibroblasts interspersed with collagen fibres which are arranged in wavy parallel bands or whorls. Fibrosarcomas are aggressive and destructive in nature. Presence of large hyperchromatic fibroblasts and several mitoses are present. Stellate or spindle-shaped cells are found in the myomas. Many strains or isolates are multipotent owing to their abilities to form tumours of different kinds such as fibrosarcomas, myxosarcomas, histiocyte sarcomas, haemangiomas and nephroblastomas etc. Rous sarcoma virus produces palpable tumours within 3 days after inoculation in chickens.	Connective tissue tumours like fibroma, fibrosarcoma, osteoma, osteogenic sarcoma and chondrosarcoma.

9. Anaplasia, metaplasia (formation of cartilage, osteoid and spindle cells), metastasis into different organs like lungs, kidneys, and spleen. Masses of altered hepatocytes formed in experimental cases of hepatocarcinoma caused by leucosis viruses.	Hepatocarcinoma
10. Portal vein of livers occluded by inward growing spindle cells from blood vessels in experimental leucosis in birds by leucosis viruses.	Endothelioma

The differences between lymphoid leucosis and Marek's disease are given in Table 7.

Table 7. Differences between Lymphoid Leucosis and Marek's Disease

LYMPHOID LEUCOSIS (LL)	MAREK'S DISEASE (MD)
1. It does not occur before 16 weeks of age and mortality occurs between 24 and 40 weeks of age. The immature Lymphoblasts in the lymphoid leucosis are pyroninophilic. B-cells are neoplastic. 2. Neural enlargement, central nervous involvement, lymphoid proliferation in the skin and feather follicles are not observed in the affected birds. 3. Nodular forms of tumours in different organs are noticed .No tumour is usually seen in skin or ovary etc.	1. It may occur as early as 6 weeks and mortality is seen from 10 to 20 weeks. Frequently noticed in paralytic form. 2. Paralysis and grey eyes are specific for MD. Nodular tumours in the skin leucosis and muscles are associated with MD. 3. Lymphoid infiltration in the nerves and cuffing around the small vessels in the white matter of cerebellum and follicular pattern of lymphoid cell infiltration in skin. 4. Premature non-specific atrophy of the bursa. The predominating medium and small lymphocytes in the tumours of Marek's disease do not stain with pyronin. T-cells are neoplastic.

Diagnosis

It is based on the symptoms , lesions and isolation of the virus from the tumours in the infected birds.Other tests like ELISA, radio immunoassay, complement fixation test and immunofluorescence are also done to confirm leucosis.

TREATMENT/MANAGEMENT

Since it is a neoplastic disease caused by a virus, there is no specific method of treating this disease. If diagnosis of leucosis complex is confirmed, the diseased birds cannot be treated and the only method is to follow genetic control or breeding programme to develop resistant strains of poultry.

Proper hygienic condition is to be maintained in the poultry farms. There should be thorough disinfection and elimination of beetles etc. from the poultry houses. No medicine is useful for treating cases of ALC or M.D. in the affected birds.

6

Fowl Pox

It is a contagious viral disease of chickens caused by a member of the genus Avipox of the family Poxviridae. The main features of the fowl pox are as under :

(1) Hyperplastic and inflammatory changes in the epidermis and feather follicles

(2) Appearance of scabs and desquamation of the degnerated epithelium. Wart-like nodules are seen on the unfeathered parts of the body

(3) Formation of the intracytoplasmic inclusions

(4) Yellowish adherent deposit is seen in the mouth. Watery or purulent discharge can be found running from the eyes and nose.

The minute coccoid components of the Bollinger bodies are called Borrel bodies. The fowl pox virus is a double stranded DNA molecule. The virus infects chickens and turkeys and produces a transient viraemia during the natural infection in fowls. Mosquitoes of the genera Culex and Aedes transmit the virus from the infected to the healthy ones. The incubation period varies from 4 to 10 days. Flock mortality can rise up to 50%.

Signs

The main changes of the fowl pox are as follows :

(1) Cutaneous lesions (resembling warts) on the head, comb, wattle, eyelids and featherless parts like legs, feet and vent in the comb form of fowl pox

(2) Diphtheritic lesions in the mouth form of fowl pox

(3) Coryza-like signs due to nasal infection

(4) No characteristic lesions in the internal organs of the affected birds

PATHOLOGY

Gross changes

Epithelial hyperplasia in the epidermis and underlying feather follicles is noticed.The nodules first appear as white foci which become yellow and also increase in size. Inflammatory and hyperaemic changes occur in such lesions and scabs are formed lasting over a week or two. The scab drops off to leave behind a smooth scar.

In the diphtheritic forms, white or opaque nodules develop on the oral mucous membrane. These nodules may coaelesce to form a yellow, cheesy and necrotic diphtheritic membrane. The inflammatory changes can spread to the infraorbital sinus and pharynx resulting in respiratory distress. There can be formation of masses of soft, yellow, diphtheritic ulcers adhering to the mucous membranes. When cheesy deposits are removed from the mucous membrane of the mouth and fauces, a raw surface is left behind it. In the oculonasal form of the fowl pox, the lesions (membranes of cheesy deposit) can obstruct the nasal cavity and lachrymal duct and infraorbital sinus. The eyelids are swollen and they stick or glue to each other due to ocular discharges. The birds with such lesions die of starvation or blindness.

Microscopic changes

The virus causes proliferation of the epidermal cells and the characteristic eosinophilic cytoplastmic inclusion bodies can be seen in the epithelial cells. The inclusion bodies may be big enough to occupy the whole cytoplasmic mass in the cells .

Diagnosis

It is based on the symptoms and lesions in the affected birds. Bollinger bodies are characteristic inclusions of the fowl pox. Agar gel precipitation test (AGPT), fluorescent antibody and ELISA tests are also useful in the diagnosis of fowl pox.

Treatment/Management

There is no specific treatment of fowl pox. Water treatment and supportive therapy (vimeral syrup and B-complex) can be given. Only control methods are reliable and the steps taken are as follows :

(1) Fowl pox vaccine can be given to chicks at the age of six weeks by cutaneous scarifications (Table 5). Chicks under six weeks of age can be given pigeon pox virus vaccine by feather follicle method. Live attenuated fowl pox strain can be used for adults and chickens. The birds which recover from fowl pox are immune and immunity in chickens can be given by vaccination from six week of age. Strong immunity gets established in fourteen days in the vaccinated birds.After about ten days of vaccination, the birds are examined for takes, which are the vaccinated birds showing swelling of feather follicles and scab formation. Pigeon pox vaccine gives protection against fowl pox.

(2) All diseased birds should be destroyed and burnt and crates and houses should be thoroughly disinfected. The birds should be kept in isolation for three weeks to be examined before mixing them with healthy flocks.

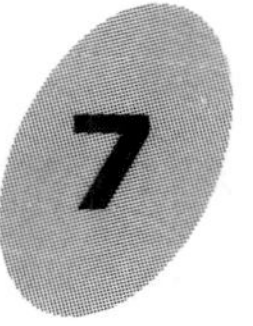

Laryngotracheitis (Infectious laryngotracheitis)

It is an acute infectious viral disease of chickens characterised by respiratory distress, depression , gasping and expectoration of bloody exudate. The changes in the tracheal mucosae include erosion, haemorrhage, swelling and oedema etc. Intranuclear inclusions are present in the epithelial cells of the tracheal mucosae of the affected birds. The laryngotracheitis virus possesses the characteristics of the herpes group of the viruses and the nucleic acid core of the virus is composed of DNA. The chickens of all ages are affected. Recovered birds act like carriers which also transmit the infection to healthy chickens. Contaminated equipment or litters or droppings can also spread infection to other birds. Incubation period varies from 6-12 days after natural exposure of birds and it varies from 2-4 days in natural exposure. The causative virus belongs to the family Herpesviridiae.

Signs

The main signs are :

(1) Nasal discharge and moist rales or whistling following coughing and gasping

(2) Marked dyspnoea and expectoration of the blood-stained mucus or slimy exudate with shreds of bright red blood

(3) Unthriftiness, reduction in egg production, watery eyes, conjunctivitis, swelling of the infraorbital sinuses, presistent nasal discharge and haemorrhagic conjuctivities can be be found in sick birds. Morbidity can be seen up to the extent of 5%. Birds recover from it in 10-14 days.

PATHOLOGY

Gross changes

The main lesions are found in the tracheal and laryngeal tissues and these are of inflammatory, degenerative and haemorrhagic types in the mucosae. Desquamated epithelial cells and blood clots are expelled by violent coughing and respiratory efforts. Inflammatory changes can also occur in the lungs and bronchi etc. The epithelium of the conjunctivae and infraorbital sinuses shows oedema and congestion.

Microscopic changes

Large masses of viral particles are present in the cytoplasm of the cells. Changes like cloudy swelling (acute cellular swelling) etc. are seen in the light microscopy. The epithelial cells enlarge, loose cilia and become oedematous. Lymphocytes, histiocytes and plasma cells infiltrate into the mucosa and submucosa of the upper respiratory tract. Haemorrhages occur in the mucosae. Cellular and mucosal degeneration are due to marked changes in the larynx and trachea. Intranuclear inclusions in the epithelial cells are noticed as early as 12 hours after infection.

Diagnosis

Symptoms and lesions are quite helpful in aiding the diagnosis of ILT. The acute signs of the disease are quite characteristic. Typical coughing, expulsion of the blood and high mortality are very marked signs of this disease. In sections of tracheal or conjunctival tissues stained with Giemsa stain, detection of intra-nuclear inclusions is quite diagnostic of laryngotracheitis. Intranuclear inclusions are quite common in the birds dead in early stages (1-5 days). Tracheal exudate or tissue suspension from affected birds can be inoculated intratracheally into healthy susceptible and immune birds to confirm diagnosis of the laryngotracheitis. ILT antibodies are detected by AGPT, indirect immunofluorescence and ELISA test.

Treatment

There is no specific treatment of ILT. Water medication and supportive (vitablend) treatment can be given.

For prophylaxis, egg propagated live virus vaccine should be administered on cloaca with brush.

Avian Encephalomyelitis (Epidemic Tremor)

It is an infectious and contagious disease of young chickens caused by a filterable virus. Mortality may be more than 50%. Affected chickens show tremors to some extent. Recovered birds, if allowed to mature, become carriers .The virus affects the central nervous system of the young fowls. Newly-hatched chickens also suffer from it. AE virus is disseminated vertically to hatched chicks from infected eggs.

Signs

The chickens (about 9 weeks old) show incoordination and sluggish movement. They develop a weakened cry, shaking of the head and quivering of the wings. Drowsiness is seen in many affected birds. There is also dullness of the eyes. Affected birds sit on their haunches or may fall to one side or walk reluctantly on hocks or shanks. When the sick birds are disturbed, there is a vibratory movement of the head.

PATHOLOGY

Gross lesions are not important but the lumbosacral enlargement of the spinal cord can be found. Microscopically, the brain and spinal cord show changes. The neurons are round in outline with swollen nuclei which assume an eccentric position. Tigrolysis or clearing of the Nissl substance is present. There is presence of bright red rounded intranuclear inclusions (equal to the size of red cells as reported (by some workers) in the affected neurons. In particularly cerebellum, the neurons disappear leaving behind themfaint pink shadows. Purkinje cells are lost in the cerebellum and gliosis develops in such areas of loss of the cells. In the pons, medulla and cerebrum, perivascular cuffing can be found. Diffuse hyperplasia of the lymphoid cells can be seen in muscular stomach, liver, pancreas and spleen etc. and increased numbers of large lymphocytes and cell debris can be found in the enlarged lymphatic foci. Infiltration of lymphocytes occurs in the muscle bundles of proventriculus is pathognomonic.

Diagnosis

The microscopic lesions like loss of neurons in the brain and lymphoid hyperplasia in the viscera is helpful in diagnosis. Neutralisation, complement fixation and haemagglutination tests are done to differentiate it from Newcastle disease.

Treatment/Management

There is no specific treatment of this viral disease in chicks, aged 1 to 4 weeks. The adult birds remain as carriers rendering the control programme as a difficult task in hatchery. The disease should be differentiated from vitamin A deficiency. The birds can be vaccinated by using a live freeze dried vaccine (Table 5). All the birds between 13-14 weeks of age should be vaccinated. The birds should have sufficient nutrition and clean environment. It is better to kill the infected birds and the dead bodies should be disposed of properly. Birds vaccinated with AE vaccine are also protected against egg drop.

Duck Hepatitis (DH)

This disease is a very acute fatal highly spreading infection of young ducklings caused by a filterable virus with characteristic lesions of hepatitis. The livers in the affected ducklings are enlarged and mottled with haemorrhages. The virus of duck hepatitis contains RNA and is a picorna virus. The virus affects only the young ducklings and the adults remain uninfected on infected farms. Chickens and turkeys are resistant to this virus. The disease spreads rapidly to susceptible ducklings in a flock. Recovered ducks may excrete virus in the faeces. In flocks up to 8 weeks after infection, morbidity in the birds will be up to 100%. Ducklings in the age group of 2-3 days or broods less than one-week old show the mortality up to 95 percent. The types of DHV are:

(1) Picornavirus (DHV I)

(2) Astrovirus (DHV II)

(3) Picornavirus (DHV III)

Signs

A very high rate of fatality is seen within 3-4 days. Stoppage of movements, partial closing of the eyes, falling of ducklings on sides, kicking spasmodically with both legs and death with heads drawn back are important signs of the disease. Death is seen within an hour after appearance of the 1st symptoms. Optisthotonus (i.e. heads stretched upwards backwards) is an important sign of the disease.

PATHOLOGY

Gross changes

The main lesions are :

(1) Enlarged livers with punctate or ecchymotic haemorrhages, frequent reddish discolouration and mottling

(2) Spleen enlarged and mottled

(3) The kidneys are swollen with congested renal blood vessels. Such lesions can develop in the young ducks on inoculation and feeding of egg-propagated virus.

Microscopic changes

It consists of necrosis of the hepatic cells and proliferation of the bile duct epithelium. The liver shows haemorrhages and inflammatory cells. The regenerated hepatic epithelium is seen in the ducklings which survive the infection.

Diagnosis

It is based on the symptoms, isolation and identification of the virus causing hepatitis in the young ducklings. The virus neutralisation test is done to identify the virus.

Treatment/Management

Serum therapy in the sick ducks with hepatitis is very useful and for this purpose, the antiserum is prepared from the recovered birds.0.5 ml of the duck hepatitis serum is injected intramuscularly in all ducklings of brood and one treatment usually suffices. It is better to immunize the whole stock. Even ducklings can be immunized with vaccine like avirulent strain of DHV. Strict isolation during the first 4-5 weeks is helpful in prevention and control of the disease.

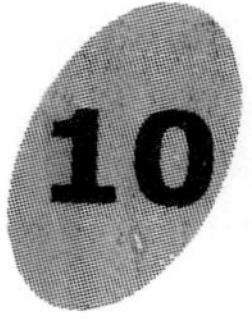

Respiratory Diseases

Mycopolasmosis (chronic respiratory disease i.e. CRD or Mg infection by *Mycoplasma gallisepticum*), Newcastle disease, infectious bronchtis, laryngotracheitis, infectious coryza (caused by *Haemphilus paragallinarum*) and aspergillosis (caused by *Aspergillus fumigatus*) constitute the respiratory diseases of chickens as a respiratory disease group. All affected flocks show symptoms like gasping, nasal discharge and coughing. In respiratory infections, an air sac lesion entity is caused and recognised by the accumulation of the exudate, thickening and discolouration of the air sacs. In chickens, M. gallisepticum causes thickening of the air sacs which get filled with exudate and the lungs become hard. This disease spreads in birds both horizontally and vertically. No signs or lesions are characteristic for Mg infection.

Infectious bronchitis is a contagious viral disease of poultry which produces lesions in the lining of trachea, bronchi and air sacs of the respiratory system. Acute respiratory disease, wheezing, coughing and death are seen in the young chickens. Low egg production and poor egg qualities are other signs of the disease. The eggs from the affected birds have thin shells and often mishapened with lumps of calcium salts deposition. The disease spreads horizontally through affected birds, air current and contaminated workmen and is caused by a RNA virus of the family Coronaviridae. There is presence of mucoid catarrhal exudate or caseous matter in the trachea and bronchi. Loss of cilia, epithelial hyperplasia and metaplasia are seen in the trachea and bronchi. The kidneys are swollen and urates are found in the tubules. In the oviducts, hypoplasia of epithelium and tubular gland and even obliteration of the lumen can be found.

Newcastle disease is a viral respiratory disease in many

countries of the world. It is a highly infectious respiratory disease marked by sneezing, rattling, coughing and signs of respiratory distress. Some birds also show nervous symptoms and mortality is very severe depending upon a particular strain of the virus. In ND-affected flocks, egg production and egg quality deteriorate very much to a low level.

The birds suffering from the respiratory disease, namely, laryngotracheitis, show characterstic symptoms and lesions. The affected birds extend heads to breathe (i.e. gasping) with production of sometimes rattling and gurgling sound. Blood is coughed up by sick birds and there is caseous material in the eyes, nose and pharynx, Diphtheritic deposit and caseous mass or clots of blood may be found in the trachea. The birds attempt to dislodge accumulations of mucus from air passages. This disease is caused by a virus which causes inflammation of the larynx and trachea. It spreads horizontally (i.e. from the contact of healthy birds with infected ones). There is a fall in egg production and the affected birds may become carriers of the virus.

Infectious coryza is also a respiratory disease caused by *Haemophilus paragallinarum*. There are discharges from the nostrils and eyes, wattles and sinuses are swollen. Transmission of the disease is horizontal (i.e. by contact with the infected birds). Drinking water contaminated with nasal discharge from infected birds infects the healthy birds i.e. mainly young chickens. It is considered as fowl equivalent of the common cold in humans.

Aspergillosis is a fungal disease affecting the respiratory system of the birds and is caused by *Aspergillus fumigatus*. Affected birds show gasping and rapid breathing. There is loss of appetite emaciation, increased thirst and appearance of some nervous symptoms in the sick birds. Cream coloured material may be found in the air sacs, syrinx, lungs and bronchi. This fungus is present in the environment and spores breathed by the chickens cause a disease called aspergillosis. Table 8 shows the main upper and lower respiratory diseases in the poultry.

There are many respiratory diseases of poultry threatening the raising of poultry in several countries and these could be divided into two groups as given in Table 8.

Table 8.

UPPER AND LOWER PARTS OF THE RESPIRATORY TRACT	DISEASES NOTICED
GROUP I Diseases affecting mainly upper respiratory tract (nose, sinus, larynx and eyes). Some birds may show lower respiratory infection at the later stages.	1. Inefectious coryza caused by *Haemophilus paragallinarum*. 2. CRD (chronic respiratory disease caused by *Mycoplasma gallisepticum*.T.A (tube agglutination) and HI test are done to diagnose it. 3. Fowl pox 4.Vitamin A deficiency. This complex respiratory disease may be seen in association with viral infections like infectious bronchitis or Newcastle disease
GROUP II Diseases affecting mainly the lower respiratory tract (trachea, bronchioles, lungs and air sacs). Some birds show upper respiratory symptoms at the later stages.	1. Gape worm infections 2. ILT. 3. Infectious bronchitis (caused by single stranded RNA virus). 4. Newcastle disease (PMV-1 infection). 5. Aspergillosis

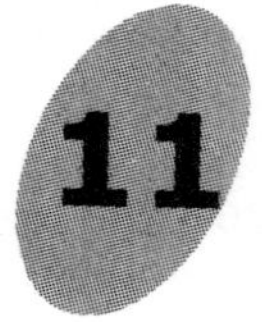

Fowl Typhoid

It is a septicaemic bacterial disease of birds (chickens and turkeys etc.) which exists in either acute or chronic form. The causal organism is called *Salmonella gallinarum*. This disease is trasmitted by the infected birds, carriers and reactors to the healthy flock. The succeeding generations in the fowls are infected through the eggs (vertical transmission). Healthy birds also get infected from contaminated attendants, clothing, crates and feeds etc. The incubation period varies from 4-5 days.

Signs

Birds (chickens and poultry) hatched from infected eggs may be moribund or dead. Somnolence, poor growth, weakness, loss of appetite and appearance of whitish material around the vent can be seen in the infected birds. Pulmonary lesions cause laboured breathing or gasping in the birds. Food consumption is reduced and the birds look droopy and ruffled with pale heads and shrunken combs. The temperature may go upto 2-5°F above the normal and mortality may vary from 10 to 50% or more. Fowl typhoid may occur severely during the period of most active egg production. The temperature in the sick birds ranges from 110 to 112°F.

PATHOLOGY

Little or no gross changes are seen in peracute cases. In the prolonged cases, swelling and redness of the liver, spleen and kidneys are seen. Greenish brown or bronze swollen livers are found in the subacute and chronic cases. Greyish white foci can be seen in the liver and myocardium and pericarditis and peritonitis arise from ruptured ova. Haemorrhagic misshapened or discoloured ova can be found. The intestines show inflammatory changes and greyish white foci are also found in the lungs, heart and gizzard. Bands of haemorrhages can be found in the proventriculus and the combs and wattles may be cyanotic in the adult.

Microscopically, the livers may show a diffuse parenchymatous hepatitis and severe fatty dystrophy. There can be lymphocytic infiltrations in such livers. Infarcts or fibrinoid necrosis and sclerosis can be found in the heart. Involution of lymphocytes can be found in the bursal of Fabricius. *S. gallinarum* is rarely localised in the joints and tendons etc.

Diagnosis

It is based on the symptoms, lesions and isolation and identification of the *S. gallinarum* from the lesions of fowl typhoid in the different organs. The liver and spleen are the organs preferred for the sake of isolating the organisms.

Treatment/Management

The treatment of fowl typhoid is like that of pullorum disease. The following steps are suggested to control the fowl typhoid (table 16). These are as follows :

(i) Maintain strict hygienic condition

(ii) Regular performance of agglutination test to remove the carriers

(iii) The reactors to the test should be removed and destroyed.

(iv) There should be disinfection of houses and small utensils etc.

(v) Birds should be given clean water.

(vi) Vaccine containing 9 R strain is available for immunization of healthy chickens against FT.

(vii) The birds can better be treated with furadentin at the dose of 0.25 gm per gallon (4.5 litre) of water. Furazolidone in the feed at a level of 0.04% for 10 days gives a very good result.

12

Avian Tuberculosis (AT)

It is a contagious disease in fowls caused by *Mycobacterium avium*. Pigeons, turkeys, geese and ducks etc. are also susceptible to it. The birds get infected through ingestion of contaminated food, water or any other contaminated material. Eggs from infected hens may contain the avian type of tubercle bacilli. Cattle may have infection with avian types of TB bacillus (*M. avium*). Humans are highly resistant to avian tuberculosis.

Signs

The main signs are :

Pallor of the comb and wattles, lameness, general weakness, anaemia and diarrhoea are noticed in the sick birds. Lameness in the birds is due to TB lesions in the joints and bones. The birds are very much emaciated and found to go light or show loss of weight. Tuberculous lesions are rarely found in birds of less than one year of age. Such lesions are noticed in old, aged or debilitated chickens which may have prominent keels due to atrophy of sternal muscles.

PATHOLOGY

Nodules and ulcers can be found on the limbs and head and the lesions are more prominent in parrots. Tuberculous lesions are found in the organs like liver, bones, marrow, lungs, spleen and intestine etc. The kidneys, ovaries and peritoneum may also contain such lesions. These lesions are as follows :

(1) White or yellowish white caseous foci (varying in size from pinhead to that of a pea) in the liver. The livers are enlarged, friable and show fatty changes.

(2) Caseous nodules in the spleen which may be also enlarged or irregular in outline. Spleen may rupture with consequent

haemorrhages.

(3) Presence of primary lesions on the outside of the intestine like raised isolated caseous (tumour like) nodules of different sizes. These nodules may form ulcers (even more than 20) in the intestines. The bacilli of tuberculosis are discharged with the faeces. The lesions are typical granulomata.

(4) Caseous pneumonia

(5) Presence of numerous small greyish white nodules in the bone marrow. Lesions-like caseous material can be seen in the joints and tendon sheaths. The surface of the joint lesions is pale-yellow in colour.

Microscopically, the tubercles consist of epithelioid cells and giant cells with usually no presence of calcification. The central area of necrosis is surrounded by cells like epithelioid cells. Fibroblasts and lymphocytes are seen at the peripheral part of the nodule. There may be rare occurrence of calcification in the lesions caused by *M. avium*.

Diagnosis

It is based on the symptoms, lesions and detection of the acid fast bacilli in the smears prepared and stained from tuberculous lesions. The tuberculin test is done by injecting tuberculin (0.05 to .01 ml) in one of the wattles which become hot, swollen and oedematous in positive reactors and the test is read 48 hours after the injection of tuberculin. The gravitation of fluid to the lower border of the swelling can be seen. The birds going light is an important sign of TB.

Prevention and Control

The treatment of tuberculosis in birds is not an economical step. Measures are taken to control and eradicate the disease. The birds are subjected to tuberculin test and the reactors are eliminated to finish the foci of infection. Repeated tests are done and reactors are removed and incinerated.

Mycobacterium avium remains alive for years in the infected soil. If the birds are allowed to occupy the infected premises, a continuing source of infection remains. It is better to dispose of all the birds (including reactors and older ones in the infected flocks) to control avian tuberculosis. The following steps are suggessted to control tuberculosis :

(1) Abandon the old equipment and new facilities are to be created.

(2) Provide proper fencing and prevent unrestricted movement of chickens.

(3) Eliminate the old flock and burn the carcasses of birds showing lesions of tuberculosis.

(4) Start a new flock (tuberculosis-fee) with a new set-up.

(5) Eliminate all swines reacting to avian and mammalian tuberculin in case of proximity of the avian flocks to pig farms. In short, the main measures are as follows :

    (a) Destroy the flocks showing reactors and disinfect the premises.

    (b) Test all the remainders and destroy the reactors.

Bacillary White Diarrhoea (BWD)

It is also called pullorum disease which is caused by *Salmonella pullorum* in fowls. The disease is chiefly associated with artificial incubation and also causes heavy mortality. *S. pullorum* produces an acute septicaemic infection in the birds. Organs like liver, lungs, yolk sac and heart blood etc. contain the organisms. These organisms are usually isolated from the ovaries of the adult birds. It chiefly infects the newly hatched chickens under 3 weeks of age. In matured birds which survive its attack, the disease exists as a chronic ovarian disease and the adults remain as its carriers. The carriers lay the infected eggs with the presence of organisms in the yolk. The chickens hatching from such infected eggs spread the infection to other susceptible chicks which get infected from contaminated particles of dust or food articles or droppings of infected chickens.The chickens are very susceptible during the 1st to 2nd days and by the fifth day, they become resistant. Contaminated incubator, brooders or attendants spread the infection to other birds. Infected cocks with orchitis also spread the infection to healthy hens and the carriers spread the infection through the eggs or droppings.

Incubation period varries from 2 to 10 days. It spreads vertically from infected hens to chicks through the eggs containing the infectious organisms.

Signs

There will be death of the embryos before hatching i.e. dead-in-shell chicks. Chickens die during the first day of hatching or shortly after hatching and the disease lasts over two to three days. Mortality may go up to 90%. Infection is harboured in the ovaries and the eggs (18% of the laid ones) contain the organisms. Diarrhoea is an important sign in the chicks hatched from infected eggs. There is also high mortality. Such birds show laboured breathing or gasp for breath.

PATHOLOGY

The main lesions are :

(1) Irregularly shaped ova are laid by the infected hens. The ova may be round, golden yellow in colour, angular, flattened, misshapened and reddish green in colour. They may be firm in consistency and attached by long stalks (i.e. pedunculated).

(2) The liver is enlarged, mottled and may show white spots.

(3) The lungs are congested and may contain yellowish white necrotic nodules.

(4) Necrotic nodules are present in the walls of heart and gizzards.

(5) Presence of catarrhal enteritis or typhlitis. The caeca are also distended with semisolid, yellow cheesy casts.

(6) Four-day-old chickens contain unabsorbed yolk-sac.

Diagnosis

It is based on the symptoms, lesions and detection of the causative organisms in the cultures. Agglutination test is done to identify the organisms and to detect the infection in adult birds. Blood is collected from suspected birds and tested against known *Salmonella pullorum* suspension. A rapid whole blood agglutination is also done. A drop of blood collected from the wing vein of the suspected birds with the help of a loop of standard size (0.02 cc) is mixed with standard antigen (0.04 cc) on a slide. In a positive reactor, the blood agglutinates within two minutes.

Treatment/Management

Drugs like furazolidone (0.04%) can be fed to infected chickens for 10 days and in case of necessity, this drug can be continued at one quarter of this level for sometime (Table 16).

This drug is available in the market with trade name of neftin. The other drug furadantin can be used at the rate of 1 lb per 160 gallon of water for 10 to 14 days.

While treating pullorum disease, it should be kept in mind that no drugs or combinations of drugs has been found to eradicate the organisms from the infected flocks. Use of sulphonamides has got demerit of interfering in feed and water intake and egg production.

Antibiotics have been tried for treating pullorum disease. The drugs are to be given in water to diseased birds with marked signs of diarrhoea to replenish the loss of water from the body (water medication).

The entire flocks should be tested for BWD every month. The positive reactors should be disposed of until the proportion of +ve reactors falls below 2%. Furazolidone at 0.04% in mash can be given. Testing is continued till all rectors are removed.

Poultry sheds or yards and utensils etc. should be clean and disinfected. If there is a need for treating cases, the reactors must be kept in strict isolation as far as possible. The birds should not be fed any egg products from infected stock. If contaminated products are fed to pigs, outbreaks of BWD can spread to healthy poultry flocks living in the close proximity to pig dwellings. The chicks should be given new boxes and flies in brooders must be controlled by spraying.

The access of sparrow to poultry farm must be prevented. Eggs should not be collected from infected birds until pullorum test clears them of infection. It has to be kept in mind that pullorum test is reliable in only sexually mature birds. The birds must not have access to poultry offal or food garbage. Testing of all flocks of birds on the farm should be carried out and new comers must react in a clean way at fortnight interval to BWD. There is no point in keeping positive or doubtful reactors for further tests and it is better to dispose of these birds. The rapid whole blood agglutination test can be used to screen the poultry farms.

Fowl Cholera (Avian Pasteurellosis)

It is an acute contagious septicaemic disease of fowls caused by *Pasteurella multocida*. There is a high mortality in fowls but the disease can also occur in subacute or chronic form. The pasteurella organisms affect fowls, geese, ducks, turkeys, pigeons and patridges etc. and the organisms are Gram negative, nonmotile and nonspore forming. The disease spreads to healthy birds by contact with infected ones through contaminatd food and drinking water or with infected droppings or saliva. The affected fowls can exist as carriers of infection, though, they themselves will appear healthy. Incubation period varies from 12 hours to 3 days. Acute or mild forms of the disease may also occur. In the acute forms, the fowls die within a few hours. The disease may last over 6 or 8 days with mortality up to 90%.

Signs

The sick birds with fowl cholera are dull, restless, and show acute illness. The comb and mucous membranes are cyanosed and discharges may escape from the beak and nostrils. There is diarrhoea in the affected birds with blood-stained loose excreta. Nasal catarrh and sinusitis may be seen in the affected birds. The wattles become swollen and oedematous. The organisms may be localised in the joints (i.e. tibio-tarsal or metapharyngeal joints) to produce lameness.

In chronic form, there is an increasing weakness, loss of weight, paleness of head and an exhausting diarrhoea. The joints in the affected birds may be swollen causing lameness in the birds. Creamy discharge from the joints or cheesy mass in the joints can be found.

PATHOLOGY

The main lesions are :

(1) Serofibrinous pericarditis and petechial haemorrhages on the epicardium along the coronary groove. The red spots on the surface of heart are due to haemorrhages in acute FC.

(2) Necrotic foci on the surface of liver. The liver may be enlarged and darkened in colour.

(3) Acute haemorrhagic enteritis. The intestinal contents are blood-tinged. The intestines are congested and haemorrhagic. There is petechiation thoughout the viscera.

(4) The lungs are congested and oedematous. Presence of pneumonia with fibrinous deposits is noticed. There may be sticky deposits in the mouth and nostrils.

(5) There are no changes in the spleen. Other visceral organs may be congested.

(6) In subacute or chronic forms of fowl cholera,the ovaries are soft, flabby and frequently show ruptures. Dried cheesy yolk-like material is present over the abdominal organs.

(7) The wattles are swollen, oedematous, shrivelled or shrunken with cheesy contents. Abscesses may be found in the joints. Presence of caseous arthritis is noticed in chronic cases.

Diagnosis

It is based on the symptoms (i.e. blood-stained diarrhoea), lesions and detection of biopolar organisms in the smears from lesions which have been stained by *Leishman's* method. Cultures are also made from the heart blood, liver and bone marrow etc. The pigeons which have been infected from materials from dead birds die within 24 hours and bipopolar rod shaped organisms can be found in the fluids or tissues. An inoculum of ground tissue can be injected into pasturella-free mice or rabbit.

TREATMENT/MANAGEMENT

All the affected birds should be treated with sulphamezathine by giving 30 ml in 4 litres of water for 2 to 3 days followed by 1/2 of the above dose for 4 days (table 16). Sulphaquinoxaline in drinking water at the dose rate of 1 ounce per gallon of water should be given. Sulcoprim, sulmet or oriprim may be used to treat sick birds.

Fowl cholera vaccine can be used to give immunity to birds. The dose is 1 ml s/c. Immunity lasts one year. Inactivated vaccine (Intervet) is available for use in the birds and contains the antigen serotype 1, 3 and 4 of *Pastuerella multocida*.

In order to control the disease, it is better to slaughter the birds and bodies should be disposed off. The birds from clean flock should be added to the existing stock. At no cost, the carrier birds should be mixed with healthy birds. Wild birds are great hazards and cause spread of infection. Perfect hygienic condition is to be maintained. All the sick birds should be disposed of in order to lessen the chance of spread among healthy birds. Pigs, dogs and cats etc. should not be allowed to enter the poultry shed to prevent the spread of infections. Infected birds should be strictly quarantined in time and poultry houses and instruments should be cleaned and disinfected before using them for fresh stock of birds.

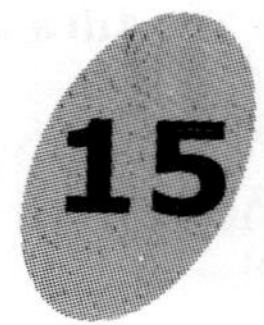

Coligranuloma (Hjärre's disease)

This disease is found in chickens and turkeys and characterised by typical granulomas or granulomatous lesions developing in the organs like caeca, liver, duodenum and mesentery. Mortality up to 25% can occur in the infected flocks. This infection is caused by mucoid coliform organisms. *E. Coli* granuloma resembles the tuberculous granuloma and these two granulomas are differentiated from each other by Ziehl-Neelsen's staining technique. Coliform organisms are non-acid fast ones. Such lesions are also produced in the susceptible birds by inoculation of ground granulomas or by intravenous inoculation of the mucoid coliform organisms.

PATHOLOGY

In the coliform infected heart, there is an oedema of the epicardium and mononuclear inflammatory cells are found in the epicardium. Heterophils can be seen passing through the intestinal epithelium. The caecum in the sick birds is enlarged and shows granulomas in their walls. Granulomas are also found in the liver in this disease. In early lesions of coligranuloma, the lesions show central mass of bacteria surrounded by heterophils, macrophages and fibroblasts. The old coliform granulomas show small necrotic areas surrounded by large giant cells. *E.coli* is found to cause serosal lesions resembling leucosis. Confluent coagulation necrosis in infection with *E. coli* can be found in the livers of the affected birds. Heterophils with a few histiocytes attempting to form gaint cells are found at the margin of the necrotic areas in the liver.

Diagnosis

It is based on the typical lesions developing in the walls of the digestive tract and liver etc. and also on isolation and identification of the coliform bacteria from the lesions. Such lesions can also be produced in the birds which are inoculated with ground material from granulomatous lesions.

Treatment/Management

It is better to find out first the drug sensitivity of the causative strain. *E. coli* is sensitive to streptomycin and chloramphenicol etc. (Table 16). A proper choice of antibiotics can be made to treat the disease. There should be increased ventiliation in the poultry house to reduce respiratory tract exposure. Faecal contamination of hatching eggs spreads the infection. The eggs should be disinfected 1-1/2-2 hours after they are laid. For this, eggs should be fumigated with 40% formaldehyde per 100 sq.feet of space.

16

Chlamydiosis(ornithosis)

It is a contagious naturally-occurring disease of non-psittacine birds caused by an organism known as *Chalamydia psittaci*. Ornithosis occurs in birds and mammals etc. Man, psittacine birds, chickens, ducks, pigeons, turkeys and pheasants are also infected by the organisms of the Genus Chlamydia. *Chlamydia psittaci* is an obligate intracellular organism. 5 to 10 percent of the affected birds die in infection with highly virulent strain, but strains of low virulence can cause mortality in less than 5% in the sick birds. Ornithosis in pigeons and ducks may have concurrent infection with salmonellae. Pigeons and ducks etc. are some of the common reservoirs of the chalamydiae.

A brief description of chalmydiosis is given below:

Chlamydiosis in ducks

Signs

(1) A severe debilitating effect and fatality in the sick birds is often seen.

(2) Trembling, imbalanced gait and cachexia in the acutely sick young ducks

(3) Presence of anorexia and diarrhoea and greenish or watery excreta

(4) Death of the birds in convulsions and mortality goes up to 30%.

PATHOLOGY

There is presence of serous or purulent discharge around the eyes and nasal orifices. Encrusts are formed in the feathers around the eyes. There is emaciation and atrophy of the muscles. Other lesions in the ducks are the following:

(1) Presence of conjunctivitis, rhinitis, bulbar atrophy and inflammation of infra-orbital sinus

(2) Atrophy of the pectoral muscles, serous or fibrinous pericarditis and hepatomegaly, splenomegaly and greyish or yellowish necrotic foci in the affected organs

Chlamydiosis in pigeons

Pigeons are the most common reservoirs of Chlamydial organisms. The young pigeons get infection through inhalation of dried excrement (nasal and intestinal) from the infected parents. Crowding and unsanitary condition expose the birds to infection.

Signs

Anorexia, unthrifty condition and diarrhoea are seen in sick pigeons. Conjunctivitis or swollen eyelids and rhinitis can also be found in them. Creaking and rattling sound are heard. Survivors become carriers. Infection with salmonellae or trichomonads causes development of signs and lesions of acute ornithosis.

PATHOLOGY

The main lesions are :

(1) Fibrinous exudate on the thickened air sacs (on the peritoneal sac), mesentery and on the epicardium.

(2) Swollen, soft and discoloured liver

(3) Enlarged, soft and dark spleen

(4) Presence of catarrhal enteritis and more urates than normal in the cloacal contents

Chlamydiosis in turkeys

Infectious dust or dried excrement from the infected turkeys spreads infection to birds in the new flocks. Chlamydiae are excreted in the droppings of ornithosis infected birds and dried excrement remains infectious for years. The organisms which have entered the body of host are engulfed by phagocytes. The organisms grow in such cells and are also released to infect other tissues. Incubation period (in experimental cases) is 5-10 days in young turkeys. Mortality may be less than 1 to 4 percent.

Signs

The affected turkeys are cachexic, anorexic and hyperthermic and excrete yellow green gelatinous droppings. There is a fall in egg production.

PATHOLOGY

Gross changes

(1) Lungs are congested. Pleural cavity contains flbrinous exudate. Dark exudate may be present in the thoracic cavity.

(2) There is thickening, congestion and coating with fibrinous exudate in the pericardium. The heart is covered with fibrinous plaques or covered with yellowish flecky exudate. There may be enlargement of the heart.

(3) The liver is enlarged, discoloured and covered with thick fibrin layer.

(4) The air sacs are thickened, discoloured and covered with fibrinous exudate.

(5) The spleen is enlarged, dark and soft. Presence of vascular congestion in the peritoneal serosae and mesentery. The mononuclear cells in the exudate contain mirocolonies of the chlamydiae.

Microscopic changes

There is presence of necrotizing and proliferative changes in the host's tissues. The lesions are more severe in young turkeys than in older turkeys. Tracheitis is characterised by extensive infiltration of mononuclear cells, lymphocytes and heterophils in the lamina propria or submucosa. Epithelioid pneumonitis is found. The lungs are congested and show infiltration of the tertiary bronchi and respiratory tubules with large mononuclear cells and fibrin. There is presence of hepatitis and diffuse diltation of sinusoids with infiltration of mononuclear cells, lymphocytes and swollen heterophils. The Kupffer cells proliferate and are filled with cell debris. Proliferative necrotic changes are found in the spleen. The vessels in the pericardium are congested. The pericardial inflammatory exudate contains fibrin, large mononuclear cells, lymphocytes and heterophils. Degenerative cellular changes are found in the kidneys. There is presence of orchitis. In the testicles, the seminiferous tubules are filled with eosinophilic exudate, fibrin, dequamated and necrotic epithelial cells and inflammatory cells can be found in the seminiferous tubules of the affected testicles. Testicular blood vessels may rupture and cause death of the birds.

Diagnosis of Chalmydiosis in birds

It is based on the symptoms, lesions, isolation and identification of Chlamydiae sp from the lesions in the body of the host. In the affected birds, there may be high circulating antibody titres of 1:64 or more. The rise in titre of circulating chlamydial antibodies is estimated to confirm the diagnosis of ornithosis.

Treatment/Management

Chickens are found to be resistant to *Chlamydia psittaci* infection. Some mortality can be seen in young birds and incidence of epizootics is very low. Turkeys are susceptible to chlamydiosis *C. psittaci* is susceptible to chloramphenicol and tetracyclines. Tetracyclines can be given in drinking water (Table 16). Turkeys can be given chlortetracyline in doses of 100 to 300 gm per tone of feed for two weeks. In pigeons, oral administration of chlortetracycline reduces mortality in epizootics and alternating period of treatment with no period of treatment helps removal of the carrier state.

Birds should be protected from inhalation of dried excrements or excreta from infected birds. Strict hygienic conditions should be maintained. The birds should not have access to infected droppings or feather dusts etc. Use of disinfected houses for birds is preferred. Birds should be added only after testing the birds or finding the birds negative for chlamydial antibody. The infected birds should be isolated. In no case, the healthy birds should be mixed with diseased birds and healthy birds should not come in contact with excretions.

There should be periodic blood testing and removal of infected birds. It is also better to have a selective breeding for resistant birds and select birds from disease-resistant groups.

17

Spirochaetosis

It is usually an acute infection of chickens and turkeys etc. caused by *Borrelia anserina* and the characteristic changes in the affected birds are as follows :

(1) Fever (up to 110^{0}F)

(2) Depression

(3) Cyanosis of head

(4) Diarrhoea

(5) Enlargement of the spleen

Argas persicus is its vector and it is a serious disease in northern India. The disease spreads to healthy birds by bites of the infected ticks. The incubation period varies from 3-8 days and the mortality may be near 100%.

PATHOLOGY

Gross lesions

These are as follows :

(1) Enlargement of the spleen and its mottling due to ecchymoses or haemorrhages

(2) The liver is also enlarged and shows haemorrhages and necrotic areas. Infarcts may be present in the liver.

(3) The kidneys are enlarged and pale. There is usually presence of mucoid enteritis in the birds. Microscopically, the reticular cells are increased in number or size in the spleen which also shows hyalinisation. Haemorrhages are found in the spleen. The liver is enlarged and there is periportal accumulation of lymphocytes, haemocytoblasts and

phagocytic cells with vacuolated cytoplasm. Fatty degeneration is present in the liver cells.

Spirochaetes are stained by silver stains in the bile capillaries and intercellular spaces. Congestion and oedema are found in the lungs. The lungs show areas of hyaline necrosis, haemorrhages and hyperplasia in the lymphoid nodules. Congestion and haemorhages are present in the kidneys. Hyaline casts can be seen in the collecting tubules. The myocardial fibres show vacuolated appearance. Congestion and haemorrhages are present in the ovaries and there is accumulation of lymphocytes around the blood vessels in the testes. Catarrhal enteritis and lymphocytic infiltration are seen in the submucosa of the intestine. Perivascular gliosis is present in the cerebrum and medulla.

Diagnosis

It is based on the symptoms, lesions and detection of the spirochaetes in the stained blood films. Droopiness, depression, stoppage of eating, cyanotic heads, ruffled feathers and greenish diarrohea are found in the birds.

TREATMENT/MANAGEMENT

Penicillin is a drug of choice and can be given to both fowls and turkeys in the doses of 5,000 to 10,000 unit/kg. body wt (table 16). Only one injection is usually sufficient.

Pronapane and Crys-4 can be used. Terramycin injectable 1 ml per bird can be given for three days. The arsenobenzon group of drugs can be used but it has got some toxic effects. Neosalvarson 30-40 mg/kg. body weight can be given parenterally.

During fever, half of the above dose should be given and should be repeated for 2 to 3 days in order to avoid ill effects.

Recovered birds are immune and chickens hatching from eggs of recovered birds have passive immunity for few weeks. Vaccine-like avianised vaccine can be used for giving solid immunity. Formaline killed vaccine can be given in a dose of 1 ml s/c to chickens at 8-10 weeks of age and the immunity lasts a year. Ticks or red mites spread infections. The birds should be kept in tick-proof house. *Argas persicuis*, a three host tick, feeds on the birds mainly at night. As the spirochaetes develop in the ticks, all stages are infective and the adults remain infective for 3 years. The tick control is needed to check the spread of spirochaetosis.

An infected adult tick can live for over two years without feed. The control of disease is a very serious problem. The ticks maintained at low temperature show reduction in infectivity and the freshly engorged infected ticks maintained at 50-60°F become sterile after sometime. The birds infested with larval ticks should be dipped in 0.5% malathion.

18

Coccidiosis

It is an important disease of poultry caused by many coccidial protozoan species which are found as intracellular parasities of the epithelium of the alimentary tract. Both asexual (one or more generations) and sexual developments happen in a single host i.e. fowl. Due to sexual life cycle, the fertilized encapsulated stage i.e. oocyst is excreted in the faeces. In coccidiosis, there are one or more asexual life cycles before excretion of coccidia as oocycsts. Coccidia have the life cycles both inside and outside the body of chickens. *Eimeria* are coccidia which contain 2 sporozoites in each of its 4 sporocysts. *Eimeria tenella* is found in the blind gut (the caeca) of fowls. It produces an acute form of the disease in baby chickens. The coccidia invade the walls of the caeca and produce extensive haemorrhages in gut. The droppings become red due to blood.

The other species of coccidia are :

(1) *Eimeria necatrix* (2) *E.acervulina* (3) *E. maxima* (4) *E. praecox* (5) *E brunetti*

E. tenella affects chickens which are 4 to 6 weeks of age. The sporozoites from the ingested sporulated oocysts are released in the gut to enter the epithelial cells of caeca. Sporozoites grow as trophozoites in caecal epithelial cells and give rise to schizonts due to repeated nuclear divisions. Segmentation of the schizonts into merozoites follows. The merozoites are released from schizonts to enter the fresh or new epithelial cells on about the 3rd day of infection.These merozoites, later, give rise to trophozoites in the epithelial cells to form 2nd generation of schizonts. Segmentation of trophozoites into merozoites in these schizonts occurs about the 5th day of infection. The asexual life cycle may continue for 3rd generation of schizonts usually after

2nd asexual stage of schizogony. The merozoites begin their sexual life cycle to form microgametes and macrogamets. These male and female gametes from zygotes due to syngamy and the zygotes so formed are passed in dropping as oocysts. Extensive damage to epithelial cells is caused by the 2nd generation of merozoites. Development of immunity in fowls is immediate in *E. tenella* infection but is delayed in *E. nectrix* infection.

Signs

In *E. tenella* infection, the birds have ruffled feather, pallor and rapid wasting of the body. Chickens (up to 2 months of age) die quickly in large numbers. The birds show droopiness and depression and droppings are haemorrhagic. When the birds survive the acute phase, oocyst production commences. Massive ingestion of oocysts by susceptible chickens causes an acute coccidiosis.

PATHOLOGY

The main lesions in *E. tenella* infection are :

(1) Blind guts (the caeca) are enlarged and filled with blood and may be plugged with yellowish cheesy substance with dark bloody areas. Excessive destruction and sloughing of the mucous membrane and submucosa is caused by 1st and 2nd generation of the schizonts.

(2) Formation of caecal plugs from the debris in the caeca

(3) Swollen mucous membrane with haemorrhages and blood-tinged exudate in the small intestine are found in *E. necatrix* infection.

Diagnosis

It is based on the symptoms and lesions and demonstration of merozoites and schizonts in the direct smears of the blood or debris in the distended caeca. Haemorrhages into mucosae and enlarged and distended caeca with discolouration are quite suggestive of acute coccidiosis. Detection of schizonts or merozontes of coccidia in the smears confirm the diagnosis. A loopful of the diluted scrapings is examined under low and high power objectives.

Treatment/Management

After coccidiosis has been confirmed by laboratory test, sulpha drugs like suphamezathine and amprolium salts etc. can be used. To control caecal coccidiosis, medicated water can be given during the period of treatment. Embazin solution can be given for water medication at the rate of 50 ml in 10 litres of water for 3 days (table 16). After a gap of two days, it is again given for 3 days. In intestinal coccidiosis, embazin can be given @ 50 ml in15 litres of water for 3 days with a break of 2 days. In short, there shoiuld be treatment of the birds for three days thrice with intervening breaks of 2 days.

Supportive treatment can also be given. Embazine and amprolium salt can also given for prophylaxis.Coccidiosis turns into a self-limiting disease, in case, the reinfection (i.e. intake of oocysts) is checked in the affected flocks. As a result, coccidial parasites are all excreted as oocysts.

19

Parasitic Diseases caused by Internal Parasites

Both the external parasites (ectoparasites) and the internal parasites (endoparasites) produce various kinds of diseases in poultry. There are several species of nematodes, trematodes and cestodes known to produce diseases in poultry. Ascaridia, caecum worms and tapeworms infect the birds. The parasitic arthropods are external parasites which include lice, mites and ticks etc. These parasites are found on the outside of the body, on the feathers and in or under the skin etc. Certain mites also occur within the body, in the air passages of the lungs and livers etc. The table 9 incorporates the names and locations of some of the aforesaid parasites affecting poultry.

The important infections caused by the nematodes, cestodes and trematodes are given below :

Diseases caused by nematodes

Oxyspiruriasis

It is caused by the eyeworm *Oxyspirura mansoni* which is found in the nictitating membrance, conjunctival sacs and nasolacrimal ducts of poultry. Embryonated eggs are laid by the parasites.

PATHOLOGY

Th worms cause opthalmia. The birds are uneasy and scratch at the eyes. The eyes are watery and show inflammatory changes. The nictating membranes are swollen and project beyond the eyelids at the corners of the eyes. The eyelids may stick together and a whiter cheesy material is found beneath them. The eye balls get destroyed due to the eye worms.

TABLE 9

Ascardia, caecum worm and tapeworms are important parasites of birds. Some of the main nematodes, cestodes, trematodes and external parasites of the poultry are given in the following table (modified after Chu, 1960)

Sl. No.	SPECIES	AVIAN HOSTS	LOCATION AND LESIONS	INTERMEDIATE HOSTS
1.	*Ascaridia galli(Nematodes)*	Chickens and turkeys	Small intestine emaciation, diarrhoea and haemorrhagic enteritis	None
2.	*Capillaria columbae*	Pigeons, chickens and turkeys	Intestine	None
3.	*Syngamus trachea*	Chickens and turkeys	Trachea. Suffocation, gasping, anemia and marked by gapes	None
4.	*Heterakis gallinaram*	Chickens and turkeys	Caecum and inflammation in caecum	None
5.	*Davainea proglot-tina (tapeworms)*	Chickens and turkeys	Doudenum Enteritis and haemorrhages produced in intestine	Slugs and snails
6.	*Taenia proglottinna (cestodes)*	*Chickens*	*Duodenitis and haemorrhages*	*Slugs and snails* (Cestodes)
7.	*Raillietina tetragona (Cestodes)*	Chickens and turkeys	Ileum, TB like nodules on the intestinal walls	Ants
8.	*Rallietina tetragona (Cestodes)*	Chickens, turkeys, guinea fowls and quails	Ileum, weight loss, fall in egg production and decreased glycogen levels in liver.	Ants
9.	*Prosthogonimus ovatus (Trematodes)*	Chickens and turkeys	Oviduct	Dragon flies
10.	*Collyriclum faba*	Chickens and turkeys	Subcutaneous cysts. Each cyst measures 4-6 mm and contains two flukes.	Probably snails and insects.
11.	*Lipeurus heterog raphus (head louse)*	Poultry	On the head. Poor health, irritation of nerve endings in the skin and blood loss in a general sense.	-

Sl. No.	SPECIES	AVIAN HOSTS	LOCATION AND LESIONS	INTERMEDIATE HOSTS
12.	*Eumenacanthus stramineus (body louse)*	Poultry	Less densely feathered parts (e.g. around the vent)	-
13.	*Menopon gallinae (shaft louse)*	Poultry	Shafts of the feathers	-
14.	*Goniocotes hologaster (fluff louse)*	Poultry	Downy feathers	-
15.	*Dermanyssus gallinae(red mites), Vectors of spiorochaetosis*	Poultry	Breeding in the birds surrounding and attacking during night	-
16.	*Cnemidocoptes mutans (scaly leg mite)*	Poultry	Found on the unfeathered portion of the leg.	-
17.	*Argas persicus (blue bug) vector for spirochaetosis)*		Found under the wings, around the vents and on the ventral surface of the body.	-

SYNGAMIASIS

This disease (also called gapes) is caused by *Syngamus trachea* in chickens, turkeys and peacocks etc. The parasites cause laboured breathing in the affected birds. The gape worm (*S. trachea*) is a red worm because of its distinguishing feature of red colour and a serious infection is caused by it in the young birds.

PATHOLOGY

The worms suffocate the birds due to obstructions caused in the trachea of the affected birds. Turkeys, poultry and pheasant chicks are very susceptible to its infection. The sick birds become weak and emaciated. The birds throw their heads forward and upward with mouth open to breath. Such convulsive shakes are attempt to dislodge the worms from the trachea to resume the normal breathing. The birds take little or no feed. The tracheal mucous membrane is inflamed and the birds cough due to irritation in the mucosae of the trachea. The inflammaory lesions are found at the point of attachment of the male worms in the tracheal mucosae and head of the male worms is found embedded in the nodular tissue. The female worms attach to the mucosae to get nourishment from the tracheal mucosae from time to time.

CROP WORM DISEASE

The nematodes occurring in the crop are called crop worms. Hair worms (*Trichuridae*) and gullet worms (*Thelazidae*) are examples of crop worms.

CAPILLARIASIS

It is a parasitic disease caused by hair worms or capillarids of the genus *Capillaria*. *Capillaria contorta* and *Capillaria annulata* are found in the oesophagus and crop. *C. obsignata* is found in the small intestine.

PATHOLOGY

The worms burrow into the crop mucose and cause its thickening and glands are also enlarged in the areas in which the worms are found. There is inflammation of the crop and oesophageal wall and in heavy infections, the surface lining of the crop is thickened, roughened and macerated. The worms are found in the sloughed off tissue. In quails and pheasants, anaemia and emaciation are noticed. The histopathological changes caused by *C. annulata* include hyperaemia, lymphocytic infiltration, formation of yellowish white nodules and enlarged lymphatic follicles in the form of nodules. Pseudomembrane containing fibrin is found over the mucosae.

In *Capillaria contorta* infection, there is thickening and inflammation in the wall of the crop and oesophagus. There can be sloughing of the mucosae and flocculent exudate can be found over the mucosae.

An infection is caused by *Capillaria obsignata* in poultry and the worm is found in the crop, oesophagus and intestine of the affected birds.

PATHOLOGY

The infected birds huddle on the ground or in some corner of the room and show symptoms of emaciation and diarrhoea. The feathers around the vent are ruffled and soiled with the excreta and the skin and visible mucous membranes are pale. Heavy infections with parasites can cause death in the birds. The caeca of the experimentally-affected chickens contains mucus, necrosed epithelial cells and lymphocytes. Haemorrhagic croupous enteritis is produced in turkeys.

GONGYLONEMIASIS

This disease in poultry is caused by *Gongylonema ingluvicola*.The worms produce burrows into the mucosae of the crop.

DISPHARYNXIASIS

This disease in poultry is caused by an ascarid called *Dispharynx nasuta*. It is found in the proventriculus of chickens, turkeys, pigeons and pheasants etc.

PATHOLOGY

The heads of worms are found buried into the mucosae and ulcers are formed in the mucosae of the proventriculus in infected chickens. The wall of the provenriculus becomes thickened and macerated and the parasites are found concealed beneath the proliferating tissue.

TETRAMERIASIS

This disease in chickens is caused by *Tetrameres americana* and the worms are found in the glandular stomach of chickens.

PATHOLOGY

The infected chickens are anaemic and emaciated. A serious catarrhal inflammation can be caused by it in the proventriculur mucosae. There is thickening of the wall of the proventriculus with even obliteration of the cavity of the glandular stomach and several worms can be found embedded in the walls of the proventriculus.

ASCARIASIS

Ascaridia galli is a common nematode found in the intestinal tract of chickens. This worms can wander up the oviduct via cloaca to be included in the developing eggs and are found at times in the eggs.

PATHOLOGY

Young chicks are most severely affected. The ascarids are found in large number in the intestinal tract. The sick birds suffer from loss of blood (anaemia), reduced blood sugar content, increased urates and retarded growth. Mortality is increased in the birds. The thymus glands of the infected chickens are shruken. Diarhoea, emaciation and droopiness are common signs in the infected chickens. The worms, if present in large numbers, block the intestines. If the fowls are infected up to the age of 3 months, these worms do a lot of damage to them.

HETERAKIASIS

This disease in chickens, turkeys, guinea fowls and pheasants etc. is caused by *Heterakis gallinarum*, which is found in the caeca of affected birds.

PATHOLOGY

These worms cause marked thickenings and inflammation of the caecal wall and are found to be carriers of the black head organism, *Histomonas meleagridis*.

They lower the resistance of the sick birds which become susceptible to many protozoal infections.

STRONGYLOIDES AVIUM INFECTION (STRONGYLOIDIASIS)

In this disease, the walls of the caeca of the fowls are thickened and the caecal contents, instead of being pasty, become thin and bloody. This worm causes serious infection in young fowls.

CESTODES (TAPEWORMS)

These are flattened ribbon-shaped worms consisting of many segments following a head region. The tapeworms grow behind the head. The oldest segments are ripe ones which are filled with eggs. These worms produce disease in fowls, turkeys, ducks, geese, pigeons, guinea fowls and many other birds. *Raillietina echnobothrida* is called nodular tapeworm. A protuberance or nodule develops in the intestinal walls at the site of attachment of each tapeworm. If no worm is found in the nodule, tuberculosis may be suspected in such fowls. This worm is called nodular tape worm. *Davinea proglottina* is one of the smallest tapeworms of poultry and is considered to be a dangerous tapeworm.

DISEASES CAUSED BY CESTODES

Davainea proglottina infection

This tapeworm infects the poultry and the infected birds become emaciated, dull and loose weight. The plumage becomes dry and ruffled. The movements in the sick birds become slow and the birds have rapid breathing. The intestinal mucous membrane becomes thickened and may be haemorrhagic and there is presence of foetid mucus in the intestine. A heavy loss due to death in poultry is caused by this tapeworm.

RAILLIETINIASIS

It is caused by many species of the family Daviaineidae in poultry. *Raillietina cesticillus* is a common tapeworm in the jejunum of poultry and causes degenerative and inflammatory changes in the intestinal villi. The level of sugar and haemoglobin falls below the normal in the affected birds.

Raillietina echinobothrida causes formation of tubercles in the intestinal wall of the infected birds. The affected birds are emaciated, become listless, lose appetite and show tendency to huddle together. They also become weak and epileptic.

Raillietina tetragona also infects poultry and quails. The birds die in heavy infection. Small nodules are found in the intestinal wall in quails. The intestinal wall is thrown into ridges of purplish colour and the intestinal mucosae slough off. The worms are found in large numbers in the intestinal lumen.

In general, birds of all ages are affected by tapeworms. The tapeworm infection causes retarded growth in the infected birds. In heavy tapeworm infections, catarrhal enteritis and diarrhoea may be seen. *Raillietina echinobothrida* forms nodules in the intestinal wall. These nodules are to be distinguished from TB nodules. Leg weakness and paralysis are found in the tapeworm infection. Capillary congestion, lymphocytic, polymorphonuclear and eosinophilic infiltration, fibrosis and proliferation in the gut are important microscopic changes associated with tapeworm infections.

DIAGNOSIS

Taeniasis is diagnosed at postmortem examination by recovering the worms from the intestine. Examination of fresh droppings for eggs or segments of the worm is not so reliable.

DISEASES CAUSED BY TREMATODES

The trematodes are parasitic organisms affecting chickens and turkeys and can be found on the skin and in the digestive and reproductive organs etc.

Collyriclum faba infection

This is a skin fluke and occurs in cutaneous cysts in the skin of chickens, turkeys and many passerine birds. The encysted flukes are mainly found in the skin around the vent and may occur on other parts of the vent. The market value of the poultry is very much affected due to these flukes.

Philophthalmus gralli infection

The flukes of this species are found in the conjunctival sacs of birds like chickens, turkeys, ducks and geese etc. The flukes attach to the conjunctivae by their suckers and produce congestion and erosions of the membrane. Blood, fluke eggs and active miracidia are found in the conjuctival fluid.

***Typhlocoelum cymbium* infection**

The fluke occurs in trachea, bronhi, air sacs and infraorbital sinus of wild water fowls, duck and goose. The flukes in the larynx and trachea may cause death due to suffocation on account of their concentration in large numbers in such vital parts of the respiratory system.

***Typhlocoelm cucumerinum* infection**

This fluke is found in the trachea of wild water fowls and also reported in the domestic duck. The flukes cause suffocation which ends in death of the birds. They are noticed in large numbers in the trachea and bronchi.

***Echinoparyphium recurvatum* infection**

This fluke has been noticed in wild water fowls and domestic birds like turkeys etc. In infected chickens, there is severe enteritis. The affected birds are emaciated, anaemic and develop weakness of legs. Cheese like exudate or mass is found in the caeca. The birds loose appetite and die. There is a fall in egg production and generalised malaise.

***Prosthognimus ovatus* infection**

This species affects the reproductive parts of birds and is very well known fluke in Asia and Europe. Affected birds show loss of appetite, normal activity and reduction in egg production. The eggs from infected birds have thin shells or no shells. The birds are emaciated and anaemic. Adhesive peritonitis is present in them. There is hyperaemia in the intestine. The intestinal mucosae have fibrinous covering . The oviduct may show rupture and albumen or yolk material can be found in the abdominal cavity. The flukes are noticed in the oviduct or egg material etc. and the birds may suffer from acute peritonitis owing to rupture in the oviduct.

Treatment/Management of worms in poultry

For controlling the worms in poultry, the faecal matter of the birds should be examined. On confirmation of the type of infestation, piprazine adipate and vermex liquid (dewormer) etc. can be used (Table 16). Taenil (I.H.) is very effective to control tapeworm infestation in poultry at 0.5 to 10% w/w mixed with feed. Control of trematodes in birds by chemical control of snail appears to be a practical approach.

For proper growth and prevention of disease and good production of eggs, the birds can be given the drugs as stated below :

Terramycin egg formula, steclin egg formula,vitablend wm forte and vimeral liquid etc.

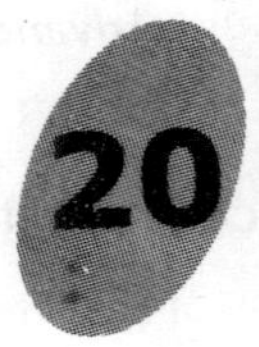

20 Parasitic Diseases caused by External Parasites

The external parasites are those arthropods which live on the outside of the body, on the feathers and in or under the skin etc. These parasites include lice, mites and ticks etc. Some arthropod parasites live in the air sac or internal organs like liver etc. Certain ectoparasites like lice eat the dead cells of the skin or its appendages. These ectoparasites draw blood or lymph through the skin of the birds (e.g. chickens, turkeys, ducks and goose etc.) infected with them. The parasites are transmitted through host contacts or may wander from bird to bird. They may even be host specific. Lice, flies, bugs and fleas etc. belong to the class *Insecta*. Mites are members of the class *Arachinida*. The names of some lices in birds are given below :

CHICKEN LICE	COMMON NAMES
Cuclotogaster heterographa	Chicken head louse
Goniocotes gallinae	Fluff louse
Lipeurus caponis	Wing louse
Menopon gallinae	Shaft louse
Menacanthus stramineus	Chicken body louse
Turkey lice	Large turkey louse
Chelopistes meleagridis	Large turkey louse
Oxylipeurus polytrapezius	Slender turkey louse
Duck and goose lice	
Trinoton anserinum	Goose body louse
Anaticola anseris	Slender goose louse
Anaticola crassicormis	Slender duck louse

Lice infestation

Lousiness (pediculosis) in birds is disgnosed by finding straw coloured lice on the skin and feathers of the birds. They measure from less than 1 mm in length to 6 mm in domestic birds. Lice eat feather products and may puncture soft quill near the bases to consume the oozing blood. They draw blood by gnawing through the layers of the skin. The lice irritate nerve endings and interfere with the rest and sleep of the birds.

Bugs

These are blood sucking parasites of the birds and their colour varies from brown to yellow or red. The bugs cause depletion of blood in the affected birds. The bites of these bugs cause swelling and itching due to injection of saliva into the wound. *Cimes lectularius* is the common bed bug which attacks man and poultry etc. They usually feed at night and bugs become engorged with blood. The other bugs are *Haematosiphon moduru* and *Oeciacus vicarius* in poultry.

Chicken mites

Dermanyssus gallinae is a chicken mite which is also called red mite or poultry mite. These mites can also attack pigeons and turkeys etc. They kill birds by extraction of blood. The birds infested with mites are anaemic and show fall in egg production. These mites look like red or blackish dots. The chicken mites spread organisms of fowl cholera, virus of equine encephalomyelitis and spirochaetes e.g. *Borrelia anserina*. *Ornithonyssus bursa* is the tropical fowl mite which attacks poultry and pigeons etc. It may harbour virus of equine encephalomeylitis. *Megninis gallinulae* is also a mite which is associated with loss of scales from the lower legs of chickens and a crusty determatitis in the head region. *Megnina ginglymura* causes a depluming itch in fowls in India. *Knemidocoptes mutans* is scaly leg mite of birds and cause lesions in the leg (unfeathered part) and comb and wattles of the birds. The mites bore tunnels into the epithelium, causes proliferation of epithelium with formation of scales and crusts in the legs. The affected birds get crippled. *Knemidocoptes gallineae* is a depluming mite. It invades the feathered parts of the epidermis of chickens and pigeons etc. The mites burrow into the shafts and cause intense irritation. The infested hosts pull out the body feathers.*Cytodites nudus* is an air sac mite found in the bronchi, lungs, air sacs and bone cavities in birds like chickens, turkeys and pheasants etc. It may cause emaciation, peritonitis, pneumonia and even obstruction of air passages. The affected birds become weak and loose weight.

Ticks

There are large parasites belonging to the superfamily *Ixodoidea* of Acarina. Ticks cause loss of blood in the infested birds with them and the sick birds may die. There is fall in egg production. The ticks also transmit disease in birds e.g. avian spirochaetosis spread by *Argas persicus*.

Argas persicus is a soft tick of fowls. Other soft ticks of fowls are :

Argas miniatus

A. radiatus

A. sanchezi

A. robertsi

A. walkerae

These soft ticks (Argasidae) are reddish brown in colour and cause loss of blood in the tick-infested birds. The birds die due to loss of blood, become emaciated, weakened and show slow growth and lowered production. The feathers are ruffled. The birds lose appetite and suffer from diarrohea. These ticks act like a limiting factor in raising poultry in many tropical countries. The soft fowl ticks transmit the pathogenic spirochaete *Borrelia anserina* in many parts of the world. Fowl ticks also transmit *Aegyptianella pullorum* and fowl cholera organism called *Pasteurella multocida*. Fowl ticks cause tick paralysis (as flaccid afebrile motor paralysis) in chickens. Hard ticks (Ixodidae) also infest poultry. Birds act like preferred hosts of larvae or nymphs of *hard ticks* like *Hyalomma* and *Amblyomma*. *Haemaphysalis hoodi* is known to kill chickens.

Treatment/Management of ECTOPARASITIC INFESTATIONS

Ticks

The litter, walls, floors, ceilings cracks or crevices in the walls or floors, outdoor runs and tree trunks should be sponged with insecticides like 3% malathion. 1% malathion can be used for spraying feed troughs (Table 17). Pestoban (I.H.) diluted with water (8 to 10 volumes) is very effective in eradicating lice, ticks, fleas and mites etc.

Mites

In order to control depluming mites (*Knemidocoptes gallinae*), the following steps can be taken for individual birds.

1. Dip the birds in a mixture of sulphur (2oz), soap (1oz) and water (1 gal). The mixture should be soaked into the skin or into the feet of birds. The birds can be dusted with 10% sulphur or 1-2oz wettable sulphur/gal as a dip.
2. Apply ointment on the affected part. The ointment consists of sulphur 1 part and petrolatum 4 parts.
3. Poultry houses must be cleaned thoroughly and disinfected before introducing new birds.

Flies

There should be proper management of the manure. Dead birds should be disposed of promptly. The littres should be kept dry and sand or new dust should be used. There should be composting of the manure and it is better to cover the manure with tarpaulin to suppress fly production etc. The manures can be treated with 0.25% dimethoate. Steps should be taken to prevent entry of flies into poultry houses. Sprays can be applied to walls, ceilings, beams and posts etc. Dry or liquid fly baits can be used to alleviate the fly problem.

Mosquitoes

There should be screening of all openings in the poultry house. Mosquitoes landing on the surfaces inside or outside of the poultry houses get killed by insecticides used to control flies. Spraying of the houses and vegetation can be done with malathion. The steps are taken to prevent breeding of mosquitoes. Swamps, ponds, pools and water-filled containers can be sprayed with malathion (Table-17) with due precautions for avoiding poisoning of birds, fishes or animals etc.

Beetles

Avoid infestation of stored grains and feed with insects or beetles. There should be fumigation of infested forages. Lesser meal worms can be controlled by spraying with 0.7% malathion.

Fleas

The infested litter should be removed. House spraying can be done to kill the immature fleas. 2% malathion can be used as spray on the floor, wall and in all cracks and crevices etc. Fresh litter should be used and it should be dusted with 4-5% malathion. Darkness, coolness, dampness and warmth are conducive for the growth of fleas.

Bugs

To kill and control the bugs, all the hiding places of bugs, cracks or crevices on the walls or floors etc. should be sprayed with 3% malathion.

Lice

Only louse-free birds should be purchased and lousy birds should not be added to fresh flocks. Malathion 2% spray can be used to kill the lice. 1% malathion dust can be used on the pigeons or in the nests to control lice.

21

Deficiencies of Minerals and Vitamins

Vitamins, amino acids and essential inorganic elements are important requirements for proper production of meat and eggs etc. in birds. All vitamins except vitamin C are required by birds. Perosis in young chickens is caused by manganese deficiency or deficiency of certain vitamins like biotin and choline etc. in the feeds. Calcium, phosphorus, magnesium, potassium, sodium and chlorine are essential inorganic elements. Manganese, iron, copper, zinc, iodine molybdenum and selenium are needed for proper growth and health of birds. Even fluorine, a consituent of the bone, is required by the birds. Vitamin E is required for preventing some diseases in birds. Chicks suffer from encephalomalacia, exudative diathesis and muscular dystrophy due to vitamin E deficiency. Addition of selenium (Se) at dietary concentrations of 0.04-0.1 part ppm prevents or even cures exudative diathesis in vitamin E deficiency. Signs of vitamin A deficiency in poultry are indicated by decreased egg production, decreased hatchability, water discharge from nosrils and eyes, sticking together of eyelids, milky white caseous material in the eyes, emaciation, weakness and ruffled feathers etc. Selenium also prevents myopathy of gizzard and heart in young turkeys. Thus, vitamin E and selenium (Se) exert a sparing effect in prevention of exudative diathesis in young chickens and myopathy of gizzard and heart in young turkeys.Deficiencies of minerals like calcium, phosphorous and manganese cause different pathlogical states in fowls. Magnesium is associated with calcium and phosphorus in the body and is also required for bone formation. The following Table 10 gives main clinical and pathological features of some important mineral deficiencies:

Table-10: Some important information in deficiencies of minerals like manganese, calcium and phosphorus.

Clinical and pathological findings	Suspected mineral deficiency
1. Perosis, gross enlargement of the tibiometatarsal joint, twisting and bending of the distal end of the tibia and metatarsus bone and slipping of the gastrocnemius tendon from its condyles. Shortening of the legs, wings and spinal column of the chicks. Occurrence of the chondrodystrophy in the embryos (i.e. globular contour of head). Affected chicks show ataxia or leg cripplings. Poor calcification of the egg shell and breaking strength of the egg shell is reduced.	Manganese deficiency
2. Rickets and formation of weak egg shells. Poor growth, weakened leg bones, and hock joints beading at the ends of the ribs. Presence of spine curve or crooked breast in the rickety birds.	Calcium and phosphorus deficiencies
3. Muscular dystrophy, exudative diathesis and encephalomalacia are seen in the affected birds.	Selenium deficiency

1. Manganese deficiency

The affected birds show slipping of gastroconemius tendon from its condyles and chondrodystrophy (deformity of bone). In this deficiency, there is hatching problem and the newly-hatched chicks may have short wings and legs with parrot beak. The birds should be given adequate amount of wheat bran and wheat product etc. The manganese to be given per lb feed is 25 mg for chickens.

2. Calcium and phosphorus deficiencies

Both calcium and phosphorus participate in bone formation. Vitamin D is required for utilisation of these two minerals. A deficiency or imbalance of calcium, phosphorus and vitamin D causes rickets in birds. Calcium deficiency causes reduction in the egg production and also formation of thin-shelled eggs.

The birds must have adequate amount of grit and limestone. The amount recommended per lb of the feed for chickens is calcium one percent and phosphorus 0.6 percent. The laying hens should be given 2.25 percent calcium and 0.75. percent phosphorus per pound of the feed.

Vitamin deficiencies or deprivations

Different diseases arise in the birds from deficiencies of vitamins. An occurrence of disease in birds due to deficiency of a single factor (i.e. a mineral or a vitamin) is quite rare but diseases due to deficiencies of multiple factors are usually found.

The important vitamin deficiencies causing diseases in the poultry are summarised as follows :

1. Hypovitaminosis A

Vitamin A becomes available to birds and animals in the form of carotene occurring with chlorophyll in the green plants. The intestinal mucosa converts one molecule of carotene into two molecules of vitamin A. Nutritional roup is a disease noticed in birds due to vitamin A deficiency. The main changes in the nutritional roup are the following :

(i) The mucous glands opening in the oesophagus or pharynx get distended with inspissated excretion. The proliferation of epithelial cells in the lining of the mucosae causes thickening and even occlusion of the glands. Squamous metaplasia and hyperkeratorsis are seen in the epithelial lining and spherical nodules or pustules like lesions (1 to 2 mm in diameter) in the epithelial linings are considered **pathognomonic** of vitamin A deficiency in birds. The affected birds show inanition, malaise, coryza and inflammatory changes in the upper respiratory tract. Ulcers can develop in the nasal passages, oesophagus and pharynx etc. in the affected chickens.

Secondary infections due to bacteria or viruses can occur in the deficient birds. Atrophy and degenerative changes occur in the respiratory mucous membrane and glandular structures. The sinuses and nasal cavities are filled with exudate. Such lesions can be found in the trachea and bronchi and nodules like particles can be found into upper part of trachea. The affected birds are emaciated and weak with ruffled feathers. There is a drop in the egg production. Hatchability is decreased with a marked mortality in eggs. Vitamin A deficiency causes retardation and suppression of endochondral bone growth. Vitamin A-deficient birds show increasd severe incidence of intestinal round worm infection . Urates are found in the kidneys of the sick birds from vitamin A deficiency. Lesions of gout can appear in the chickens ailing from hypovitaminosis A.

Treatment/Management

The birds showing symptoms and lesions of vitamin A deficiency should be given adequate quantity of burseem and other greens, fishoil and vitamin A concentrate etc. The different doses in the chickens are as follows:

(i) Chicks 3,000 I.U.

(ii) Growing pullets 3,000-4,000 I.U.

(iii) Laying hens 4,000 I.U.

(iv) Turkeys 4,000 I.U.

The above dose rate of vitamin A has been given in view of per lb of feed preparation. However, vitamin A preparation can be given at the level of 5,000 I.U. per lb of ration on a general basis.

2. Biotin deficiency

Affected birds show determatitis of feet, congenital perosis, ataxia and skeletal deformities. Hatching problems arise and the chick embryos show reduction in size and parrot beaks.

Treatment/Management

The birds must have sufficient amount of fresh greens and molasses etc. They should also be given grain products. The amount of vitamin recommended per lb of feed is as follows :

(i) Chicks -50 micrograms

(ii) Breeding hens - 70 micrograms

3. Pantothenic acid deficiency

It is the vitamin part of the Coenzyme A which takes part in several reactions of fat, protein and carbohydrate metabolism. This is also required for acetylation of choline to form acetylcholine. Its deficiency in the body causes subcutaneous haemorhages and oedema in the developing chick embryo. Dermatitis, broken feathers, perosis, retardation in growth and mortality are seen in chicks. The chicks are emaciated with crusty scab like lesions in the corners of the mouth. Scabs develop on the margins of the eyelids which are stuck together by viscus exudate . Sloughing and keratinisation of the epithelium of skin are noticed. Small cracks are seen at the outer layer of the skin betwen the toes. Puslike exudate is found in the mouth. There is presence of greyish white exudate in the proventriculus. Hypertrophy of liver which becomes faint or dirty yellow in colour. Myelin degeneration is found in the myelinated fibres of the spinal cord.

Treatment/Management

The birds should be given whey, yeast, liver meal, rice bran and molasses. The amount recommended per of 1b feed is as follows :

(i)	Chicks, growers and laying hens	5-7 mg
(ii)	Breeding hens	5 mg
(iii)	Turkeys	7 mg

4. Vitamin K deficiency

It is needed for synthesis of prothrombin which participates in clotting of blood. Due to vitamin K deficiency, chicks show anaemia and loss of blood etc. Disturbance in the blood clotting and determination of prothrombin time help in its diagnosis.

Treatment/Management

The birds should be given green grasses and cereals etc. The amount of vitamin K per 1b feed is 0.6 to 1.5 mg. The affected birds with vitamin K deficiency show haemorrages in the legs, breast and also failure of blood clotting.

5. Folic acid deficiency

Folic acid takes part in nucleic acid metabolism and is required for formation of nucleoproteins. Folic acid deficient birds show poor growth, poor feathering, anaemia and perosis. Embryonic mortality arises from its deficiency. Cervical paralysis is present in the affected poultry. Macrocytic anaemia is seen in the chicks suffering from folic acid deficiency.

Treatment/Management

The affected birds suffer from deformed beak and drooping of wings. The birds should be given adequate amount of green and wheat bran etc. 0.3-0.5 mg of folic acid per 1b of feed can be given to sick birds.

6. Vitamin E deficiency

Vitamin E-deficient chicks show encephalomalacia, exudative diathesis and musular dystrophy. Enlarged hocks and dystrophy of the gizzard musculature are found in the affected turkeys.

There is a reduction in hatchability in chickens and turkeys. Ataxia, backward or downward retraction of head and incordination are seen in the vitamin E-deficient chicks. The cerebrum is soft and swollen and haemorrhages are found on the cerebellum and the convolutions are flattened. Oedema of the subcutaenous tissue and abnormal permeability of the capillary walls are seen in exudative diathesis of chickens. Distension of the pericardium is found in the dead birds. The affected muscles in the vitamin E deficient birds show hyaline degeneration. Adequate amount of vitamin E with selenium supplementation produces good result in selenium deficiency. Sections of bony lesions reveal increased osteoid and the columns of chondrocytes in the degenerated hypertrophic thickened epiphyseal plate which may be invaded by metaphyseal blood vessels. Irregular columns of cartilage cells and elongated epiphyseal vessels are noticed in rickets.

Treatment/Management

The birds should be given wheat germ oil, soyabean oil and grain etc. The vitamin E is recommended per lb of poultry feed in the doses of 13-15 I.U.

7.Vitamin D deficiency

Vitamin D is needed for proper metabolism of calcium and phosphorus. Vitamin D deficient birds suffer from rickets. Thin shelled or soft shelled eggs are found in deficient birds. The beak, claws and keel become soft and pliable. There is also bending of the sternum or spinal column. In general, bones become weak. On postmortem examinations, the bones are found to be soft and also break with little effort. Skeletal distortions are found. Renal damage (dystrophic calcification) is found in hypervitaminosis D.

Treatment/Management

The birds showing rickets and beaded ribs should be given fishoil, irradiated animal steroid or Vitamin D3. The formula for the preparation of poultry feeds containing vitamin D per lb feed is given below :

Baby chicks or growers	-250-500 ICU (International chick unit)
Hens	-400 ICU
Turkeys	-600 ICU

Sunlight is beneficial for the vitamin D-deficient birds.

8. Hypovitaminosis B1

In vitamin B1 (thiamin) deficiency, the affected birds show anorexia, paralysis of muscles, loss of weight, ruffled feathers, drooping of wings and unsteady gait. The birds sit on their flexed legs and draw back the heads in the star-gazing position. Atrophy of the testes is seen. There is polyneuritis and oedema of the skin.

Treatment/Management

Grains and oilcake meal should be given to birds. 1 mg of thiamin per lb of feed can be given to sick birds.

9. Pyridoxine (Vitamin B6) deficiency

Depressed appetite, poor growth, perosis and nervous symptoms are seen in the pyridoxin-deficient birds. Jerky movements and spasmodic convulsions are noticed in the sick birds. Loss of weight, decreased feed consumption and reduction in the egg production and hatchability are found in the adult birds.

Treatment/Management

The bird should be fed cereal grains, yeast, alfalfa meal and animal products etc. The vitamin B6 recommended per lb of feed is as follows :

Chicks 2 mg

Poults 2 mg

10. Vitamin B2 (riboflavin) deficiency

The birds suffering from riboflavin deficiency are weak and emaciated with poor growth and the birds suffer from diarrhoea between the 1st and 2nd week. The affected birds walk upon their hocks with the aid of their wings when they are forced to move. The toes are curled inward during walking and resting and the birds are seen in a resting position (curled toe paralysis). There is often drooping of the wings in the affected chickens. Dry and harsh skin with atrophied and flabby leg muscles is seen.

The egg production is decreased and enhanced embryonic mortality is noticed. The liver is increased in size and the fat content is increased in liver. There is swelling and softening of sciatic and brachial nerves in chickens. The myelin sheaths of the peripheral nerves show degenerative changes and the axis cylinder may undergo swelling and fragmentation. Schwann cell proliferation, myelin changes, gliosis and chromatolysis are found in the spinal cord. Muscular degeneration is noticed in riboflavin deficiency in chickens.

Treatment/Management

The birds suffering from Vitamin B2 deficiency show curled toe paralysis with atrophy of leg muscles. The birds should get adequate quantity of milk product, fresh grain, yeast and fermentation products etc. The dose of riboflavin in feed is as follows.

2 mgs of vitamin is given to starting chicks, growing chicks and laying hens per lb of the feed. 3 mg of the vitamin is to be given to starting poults and breeding turkeys per lb of the feed preparation.

11. Vitamin B12 deficiency (cyanocobalamin)

Vitamin B12 deficient birds show slow growth, poor feed utilisation and reduced hatchability. Perosis may also occur in the deficient birds. There is high mortality of embryos with peak of mortality on the 17th day of hatching. Leg muscles show atrophy and haemorrhages in the embryos are seen.

Treatment/Management

Fish meal, milk product, animal proteins and dried cow manure may be given to birds, 3-6 micro g per lb of feed is the recommended amount of vitamin B12 for sick birds.

12. Choline deficiency

Its deficiency causes perosis. There are pinpoint haemorrhages and puffiness about the hock joint. Deformity in the tendon of Achilles is seen and the tendon slips from its condyles. The livers of the deficient birds show abnormal fat content.

Treatment/Management

Yeast, fish meal, oil cake, meal and synthetic choline can be given to birds. The amount recommended per lb of feed is as follows :

Chicks - 700 mg.

Poults - 900 mg.

Diagnosis of Poultry Diseases

Some lesions in different diseases are suggestive of certain diseases. In fact, there are a very few pathological changes which can be considered as specific ones for a single disease. The diseases in the birds or animals are represented by a variety of pathological and clinical features. A definite diagnosis is always done with the help of bacteriological, virological, parasitological and other laboratory tests. A disease in a fowl can be considered as a flock disease. This is because many chickens show more or less similar signs and lesions in a flock at a time. Pathognomonic lesions are quite specific tissue changes as diagnostic tools of poultry diseases (table11).

Table 11. Pathognomonic lesions in some poultry diseases

Diseases	Lesions
1. Ranikhet disease (RD)	Petechiae or haemorrhages at the junctions of proventriculus with the oesophagus and gizzard and in small intestine, caecal tonsils etc in the infected dead birds.
2. Infections bursal disease (IBD)	Enlarged cream coloured bursa of Fabricius, gelatinous yellowish transudate on the serosal surface, oedema, hyperaemia, ecchymotic haemorrhages on the mucosal surface of the bursa and haemorrhages throughout the bursa in some cases.
3. Avian encephaloymelitis (AE)	Dense lymphocytic foci or aggregates in the muscular wall of proventriculus, and gliosis in the molecular layer of the cerebellum, brain stem and optic lobes et

Diseases	Lesions
4. Histomoniasis (*Histomonas meleagridis*) infection affecting turkeys or suitable avian hosts	Circular depressed areas of necrosis (about 1cm in diameter) i.e. circumscribed lesions with raised rims.
5. Vitamin A deficiency	Spherical nodules (about 1 to 2 mm in diameter over the pharyngeal and oesophageal mucosae, squamous metaplasia and hyperkeratosis in the ephithelial linings of ducts of mucus glands opening in the pharynx and oesophagus.

The Table (modified after Chu, 1960) giving information about related causes, clinical and pathological changes and diseases to be suspected are given below :

Table 12. Causes, signs and lesions in different diseases

Possible causes	Clinical and pathological findings	Disease conditions
Vitamin A deficiency. High intake of protein rich feed or protein, impaired excretory function of the kidneys due to poisons or toxic material. Dehydration is a common cause of visceral gout in poultry.	1(a) Excess of uric acid in the blood. Deposit of urates on the serous surface of liver, pericardium, abdominal air sac and in the tubules of kidneys and joints etc. Renal lesions, white pasting of cloaca, dilated ureters and deposits of urates on heart, liver and lungs etc.	Kinds of gout (a) Visceral gout.
	1(b) Pain and acute inflammatory changes in the joints and deposits of white chalky materials (called tophi) in the articular and periarticular tissues of the joint. Pain arising from sharp crystals of chalky deposits.	(b)Articular gout

Possible causes	Clinical and pathological findings	Disease conditions
Intakę of large quantity of fibrous and bulky material, ground straws and sawdust.	Over distension of crop. The crops are dilated, flabby and filled with fowl-smelling feeding stuff or foreign materils.	2. Crop impaction.
Uncertain causes, change of ration or a fresh supply of feed on feeding of a new wheat and nephritis due to metabolic disorder.	Cyanosis of head (blue comb). Distension of crop and watery diarrhoea. Focal necrosis and haemorrhages of liver, degeneration of breast muscle and haemorrhages on the serous membrane. Nephritis (uraemic). Presence of leucocytosis.	3. Blue comb pullet disease.

Table 13. Signs and Lesions In Different Diseases

CLINICAL AND PATHOLOGICAL SIGNS IN THE DISEASED BIRDS	DISEASES SUSPECTED
(i) Coryza syndrome Nasal catarrh, conjunctivitis and sinusitis and presence of caseous mass	1.. Infectious coryza (*Haemophilus para gallinarum*). 2. CRD (*Mycoplasma gallisepticum* infection) 3. Fowl pox. Pox lesions are usually found on the mouth, larynx and skin. 4. Vitamin A deficiency Nodules usually present on the oesophagus and crop. The kidneys contain urates.
(ii) Tracheitis, bronchitis (with or without airsac involvement or coryza).	1. Infectious laryngotracheitis 2. Newcastle disease. 3. Infectious bronchitis 4. Aspergillosis 5. Fowl pox 6. Fowl plague 7. Pasteurellosis 8. CRD (*M/ gallisepticum* infection)

CLINICAL AND PATHOLOGICAL SIGNS IN THE DISEASED BIRDS	DISEASES SUSPECTED
(iii) Airsac infections, presence of thickening of thoracic and abdominal airsacs with exudate of caseated mass.	1. Secondary complications due to Newcastle disease 2. Infectious bronchitis 3. Coliform infection 4. Peritonitis 5. Aspergillosis
(iv) Petechial haemorrhages on the organs like heart, pericardium and peritoneum.	1. Haemorrhagic syndrome 2. Fowl plague 3. Newcastle disease 4. Pasteurellosis 5. Spirochaetosis 7. *Aegyptianella pullorum* infection (with enlarged spleen and liver) 8. Erysipelas
(v) Enlarged liver and spleen	1. Spirochaetosis (spleen mottled) 2. *Aegyptianella pullorum* infection 3. Fowl typhoid (bronze coloured liver) 4. Erythroleucosis (bright red liver and spleen) 5. Lymphomatosis (with white nodules) 6. Myeloid leucosis 7. Tuberculosis (caseated nodules raised over the surface of liver and nodules in the bone marrow) 8. Black head (ulcerations with caseated plug in the caecum) 9. Ornithosis 10. Erysipelas (*Erysiplothrix rhusiopathiae* infection)
(vi) Haemorrhagic ovaries	1. Egg peritonitis 2. Spirochaetosis 3. Fowl typhoid 4. Newcastle disease 5. Pullorum disease

CLINICAL AND PATHOLOGICAL SIGNS IN THE DISEASED BIRDS	DISEASES SUSPECTED
(vii) Degenerated ovaries	1. Egg peritonitis 2. Fowl typhoid 3. Spirochaetosis 4. Pullet disease
(viii) Unabsorbed yolk in chicks	1. Chills 2. Pullorum disease 3. Mushy chick disease
(ix) Caseous exudate in the mouth or scab like lesions in the corner of the mouth and eyes.	1. Fowl pox 2. Vitamin A deficiency 3. Pantothenic acid and biotin deficiencies 4. Thrush 5. Riboflavin deficiency in turkeys
(x) Pseudomembranous inflammation and ulcerartion in the oesophagus and crop.	1. Turkey or pigeon pox 2. Thrush (moniliasis) 3. *Trichomonas* spp. infection
(xi) Haemorrhages in the proventriculus	1. Ranikhet disease 2. Fowl plague 3. Spirochaetosis 4. Sulphadrugs poisoning (with subcutaneous haemorrhages) 5. Gumboro disease 6. Mouldy corn poisoning
(xii) Haemorrhages in small intestine	1. Spirochaetosis 2. Newcastle disease 3. Fowl plague 4. Intestinal coccidiosis 5. Pasteurellosis 6. Sulpha drug poisoning 7. Fowl typhoid 8. Haemorrhagic syndrome
(xiii) Haemorrhages in the caecum	1. Coccidiosis 2. Black head (with ulcers in the liver)

CLINICAL AND PATHOLOGICAL SIGNS IN THE DISEASED BIRDS	DISEASES SUSPECTED
(xiv) Haemorrhages in proventriculus and caecal tonsils. Haemorrhagic necrotic enteritis.	1. Ranikhet disease
(xv) Nervous symptoms like incoordination and paralysis etc.	1. New castle disease or vaccination reaction with respiratory or other symptoms 2. Fowl paralysis (with enlarged bracheal and sciatic nerves (or plexuses) 3. Avian encephalomyelitis (with encephalomyelitis and muscular dystrophy) 4. Vitamin deficiency (with polyneuritis in B1 deficiency and curlytoes in Vitamin B2 deficiency) 5. Vitamin E deficiency (oedema, haemorrhage and necrosis in brain) 6. Overheating marked by acute congestion of lungs.
(xvi) Weakness of legs	1. Fowl paralysis (MD) 2. Vitamin D deficiency (soft bone) 3. Riboflavin deficiency (curlytoes) 4. Thiamin deficiency 5. Choline deficiency 6. Arthritis or synovitis 7. Manganese deficiency
(xvii) Erosions in gizzards	1. Nutritional deficiency
(xviii) Enlarged nerves	1. Fowl paralysis (MD)
(xix) Nodules in small intestine	1. Tuberculosis 2. Tapeworm infection 3. Leucosis complex (ALC)
(xx) Nodules in lungs	1. Aspergillois 2. Pullorum disease 3. Leucosis complex (ALC)

CLINICAL AND PATHOLOGICAL SIGNS IN THE DISEASED BIRDS	DISEASES SUSPECTED
(xxi) Nephritis	1. Visceral gout 2. Vitamin A deficiency 3. Pullet disease 4. Chills 5. Salt poisoning 6. Metabolic disturbances
(xxii) Swollen head and wattles	1. Head injuries 2. Chronic pasteurellosis 3. Coryza 4. Fowl pox 5. Emphysema
(xxiii) Distended gall bladder	1. Enteritis 2. Vitamin A deficiency 3. Pullorum disease 4. Chills in chickens 5. Fowl typhoid.
(xxiv) Watery blood	1. Spirochaetosis 2. Malnutrition 3. Other blood parasites
(xxv) Clear yellow or blood tinged fluid in the thorax and abdominal spaces. Hypertrophy or enlargement of right ventricle and enlarged and congested liver.	1. Ascites cum right ventricular failure (ARVF). Such condition can arise from pulmonary hypertension, Nacl poisoning and chills etc.
(xxvi) Bursa of Fabricius enlarged, oedmatous and haemorrhagic with cream coloured appearance. Petechiae can be found in the pectoral and thigh muscles. Such lesions in the bursa are pathognomonic for IBD.	1. Gumboro disease (IBD)
(xxvii) Perihepatitis and pericarditis	1. Ornithosis and coliform infection.

While diagnosing avian diseases, serlogical tests are required in suspected cases of *S. pullorum* and New castle disease (e.g.HI test in RD). Infectious bronchitis and many other virus infections require serum netralisation tests for diagnosis. Routine parasitological examination is done in the cases of coccidiosis (smear of exudate from caecum and small intestine) and external parasitic infections (ticks, lice and mites etc.). Histopathological examination is done to diagnose diseases like avian leucosis complex (ALC), avian encephalomyelitis and other nervous diseases and intestinal coccidiosis etc. The following clinical and pathological signs are helpful in the diagnosis of certain poultry diseases (Table 14)

Table 14. Signs, Lesions and Diseases Suspected

Clinical and pathological signs	Diseases suspected
Presence of injuries around the cloaca and on the head and back, overcrowding, dietary deficiencies of proteins, salts and grains etc.	1. Cannibalism (head or feather pecking)
The chicks huddle together and there is pasting up of the cloaca. In the birds examined after death, unabsorbed yolk, distended gall bladder, congested lungs, nephritis, empty crop, dirty brown fibrous material in the gizzard and undigested food in the intestine are found. Failure of heating system or wind draft in the room of the chickens cause such signs and lesions.	2. Chills in chickens
Sweating, wet feathers, respiratory trouble, nervous symptoms (retraction of the head etc.). Acute congestion of lungs, pneumonia, congestion and haemorrhages in brain are found in the affected birds. The aforesaid conditions are caused by overcrowding, fault in the heating system and poor ventilation etc. Fall in egg production, small eggs being laid by birds, reduced appetite, panting, increased thirst, haemorrhages on liver and crooked appearance of the breast muscles.	3. Heat stroke

Clinical and pathological signs	Diseases suspected
Cannibalism, sweating, and wet feathering and keratoconjuctivitis due to NH3 (ammonia) accumulation in the air. The symptoms like respiratory distress are seen. Congestion of lungs and other internal organs. Such conditions are caused by faulty ventilation and lack of adequate space to each bird (i.e. overcrowding).	4. Respiratory diseases
Respiratory distress, congestion, pneumonia, presence of greyish cheesy exudate or nodules in the bronchi, lungs and air sacs etc. Such signs or lesions are more common in pullets than in chickens and are caused by moldy feed or bedding, dirty moldy water troughs and feeders etc. Microscopically, nodular lesions in the lungs reveal caseation necrosis, ephithelioid cells, giant cells of foreign body types and septate branching fungi.	5. Aspergillosis (Brooder pneumonia)
Difficult respiration, increased thirst, generalised oedema and musclar weakness. Postmortem examination of dead birds shows inflammation of the mucous membrane of the crop, proventriculus and intestine, general oedema, pericarditis and ascites, congestion and blood stained appearance of organs like muscle, kidneys and lungs etc.	6. Sodium chloride poisoning
Slow growth, lower egg production, cannibalism, watery excreta, poor feed conversion. Nervous signs (like tatanus) and fall on the ground with the legs streched from sharp noises.	7. Sodium chloride deficiency

Clinical and pathological signs	Diseases suspected
Poor growth, ruffled feathers, lack of yellow pigments in the shanks or beaks, lachrymation and presence of cheesy material under the eyelids. Coryza syndrome, pustules in mouth, oesophagus, crop and respiratory tract. Deposition of urates in the tubules of the kidneys, ureters, cloaca and on heart, pericardium, omentum, liver and spleen etc. Drop in egg production, decrease in hatchability and high mortality of chickens during the first two weeks of life.	8. Vitamin A deficiency
Leg weakness, retardation of growth, low egg production, low hatchability and thin or soft-shelled eggs.	9. Vitamin B deficiency
Soft rubbery and pliable bone and beaks, distortion of skeletons, bending of sternum (crooked sternum) and spinal column and enlarged hocks. Tendency to sit on the hock and reluctance to move. An osseous disease of young growing birds.	10. Rickets
Encephalomalacia in chickens, myopathy in ducklings (occurring between 2-4 weeks). Ataxia (lack of cordination), retaraction of head, lateral twisting and forced movement, oedema, haemorrhages and necrosis in cerebellum and cerebrum, flattened convolutions and poor hatchability in breedings hens.	11. Vitamin E deficiency
Polyneuritis with nervous symptoms like retraction of head, opisthotonus, paralysis of muscles, weakness of the legs, unsteady gait and drooping wings.	12. Thiamine (Vitamin B1) or antineurin deficiency.

Clinical and pathological signs	Diseases suspected
Increased embroynic mortality (dead in shell chicks) with curly toes. Curled toe paralysis in the chicks or pullets, sitting on their hocks with aid of wings, atrophy of leg muscle, enlarged eyelids and mouth. Degeneration of myelin sheath.The hatched chicks are dwarfed, oedemaous and show clubbed down resulting from failure of the down feathers to rupture the sheath.	13. Riboflavin (Vitamin B2) deficiency
Retarded and rough feather growth, loss of feathers from the head, sloughing and keratinzing epithelium of the skin, appearance of cracks and fissures between the toes, cornified and wart-like protuberance on the balls of the feet. Egg production and hatchability affected. Crusty scab like lesions in the corner of the mouth and margins of the eyelids and pus like substance in the mouth. Embryos oedematous and haemorrhagic.	14. Pantothenic acid (antidermatitis factor) deficiency
Presence of dermatitis, poor hatchability and perosis. Chrondrodystrophy and deformed parrot beak are seen.	15. Biotin deficiency
Flattening of tibiometatarsal joint, twisting and bowing of metatarsal, slipped tendon and poor growth.	16. Choline deficiency
Nervous symptoms, spasmodic convulsions and jerky movement of the legs. Presence of demyelination and chondrodystrophy.	17. Pyridoxine (Vitamin B6) deficiency
Haemorrhages on the legs, breast and wings and failure of the blood to clot due to decrease in thrombin content.	18. Vitamin K deficiency

Clinical and pathological signs	Diseases suspected
High mortality, kidney hypertrophy, increase of non-protein nitrogen in the blood, high mortality of embryos, the peak of mortality at 16th day of hatching, myopathy of legs, haemorrhages of the embryos and allantois and low feed consumption. Reduced size, perosis, oedema and fatty liver in vitamin B12 deficient embryos.	19. Vitamin B12 deficiency
Nodules on the oesophagus, caseous exudate in the eyes and urates in the kidneys.	20. Respiratory diseases (a) Vitamin A deficiency
Short incubation period (1 to 2 days) with favourable response to sulpha drugs Coryza syndrome.	(b) *Haemophilus paragallinarum* infection
Long incubation period (5 to 21 days) and prolonged course. No response to sulpha drug treatment.	(c) CRD i.e. Mycoplasmosis (MG infection)
Pox lesions on wattles, eyelids and mouths and the combs. Diphtheritic or necrotic material in the oral cavity.	(d) Fowl pox
Pseudomembranous or haemorrhagic tracheitis, severe gasping and high mortality. The birds extend the head to breathe and blood is coughed up.	(e) Infectious laryngotracheitis (ILT)
Short incubation (1 to 3 days), brief course and low mortality. Presence of sneezing and gasping. Catarrhal tracheitis and rhinitis with cheesy plugs in the bronchi.	(f) Infectious bronchitis(IB)
Yellow white nodules in bronchioles and lungs saucer-shaped lesions with depressed centres on the air sacs. Greenish moudly appearance of lesions.	(g) Aspergillosis (brooder pneumonia)

Clinical and pathological signs	**Diseases suspected**
Sneezing, gasping, presence of nervous symptoms. High mortality, sudden outbreak, presence of haemorrhages or petechiae on heart, proventriculus intestine and caecal tonsils etc.	(h) Newcastle disease(Ranikhet disease)
Inflamed yolk sac and coagulated or turbid yolk	21. Omphalitis (caused by factors like *E. coli*, *Pseudomonas* spp. and staphylococci and *Salmonella* spp. etc.

23

Infectious Bronchitis

It is an acute contagious viral disease of chickens. The causative agent is an avian infectious bronchitis virus (IBV) of the genus *Coronavirus*. Turkey IB virus also belongs to this genus.The characteristic features of this disease are tracheal rales, coughing and sneezing, serous, catarrhal or caseous exudate in the trachea, nasal passage and sinuses. This disease is a very severe infection in baby chicks. Chickens of all ages are susceptible to IBV. The incubation period of IB is 18-36 hours. Mortality in the affected birds may reach up to 25 percent.

Signs

The main signs are as follows:

1. Gasping, coughing, sneezing, tracheal rales, nasal discharge, wet eyes and swollen sinuses in the infected chicks
2. Depression and huddling under a heat source, reduction in weight gain and feed consumption are seen in chicks infected with the coronaviruses.
3. Ruffled feathers , wet droppings and increased drinking of water are seen in the recovered birds from infection of nephropathic coronaviruses. Urolithiasis is noticed in such infected flocks.
4. Decreased egg production and respiratory signs in laying flocks infected with coronaviruses.

The main gross lesions are:

1. Serous or caseous exudate in the trachea and nasal passages etc.
2. Cloudy appearance of air sac and yellow caseous exudate are seen in the air sacs. Caseous plug is also noticed in the

lower trachea of bronchi of the affected chicks.

3. Swollen pale kidneys along with tubules and ureters distended with urates in the chickens infected with coronaviruses.

4. Presence of fluid yolk material in the abdominal cavity of layers. Nonpatent and hypoglandular oviducts are found in chicks infected with IBV.

The main histopathological lesions are:

1. Stained sections of trachea reveal oedematous trachea and cilia in the trachea are lost and epithelial cells slough off. Heterophils and lymphocytes may infiltrate into the trachea. Epithelial regeneration is also noticed in the trachea and lamina propria of tracheal muscosa shows several germinal centres and infiltration of lymphocytes.

2. Oedema, desquamation of epithelial cells and proliferation of fibroblasts are noticed in the infected sacs which also contain caseous exudate.

3. The kidneys show interstitial nephritis due to IBV infection. Marked infiltration of heterophils in the interstitium and granular degeneration, vacuolation and desquamation of the tubular epithelium are the main histological lesions. Focal areas of necrosis and regeneration of tubular epithelium are also seen in the infected kidneys.

4. Urolithiasis is noticed in affected atrophic kidneys. Ureters in the kidneys are distended with urates or calculi of urates in IBV infection.

Diagnosis

It is based on the symptoms, lesions and isolation of the virus. Immunofluroscence helps detection of IBV antigen in tissue sections or smears. It should be differentiated from ND, ILT and IC (infectious coryza) etc.

Management/Treatment

Chicks recovered from infection with one IBV strain are susceptible to another IBV strain.There is no specific therapy for IBV infection. Provide additional heat to protect chicks from cold. Overcrowding is to be avoided and the chicks are given adequate quantity of feeds. Antibiotics are used to protect birds form air sacculitis. Isolate the infected birds. Poultry houses should be cleaned and then repopulated with day-old chicks. Avoid air-borne infections.

Both live and inactivated viruses are used to provide immunity against IBV infection. Live vaccine of IBV with Newcastle disease virus is used to provide immunity. The attenuated Massachusetts strain is a safe vaccine for chickens. One drop of vaccine is administered in each eye.

A vaccination schedule against IBV infection is as follows:

IB Vaccine	**Age of chickens**
1. Primary	4 weeks.
2. Booster	14 to 16 weeks

24

Influenza (Avian Influenza or Bird Flu)

It is an infectious disease or a disease syndrome in poultry caused by type A influenza virus of the family Orthomyxoviridae. Influenza viruses infect both birds and humans.Outbreaks of avian influenza cause a considerable loss to poultry industry and this virus also infects turkeys, chickens, guinea fowls, ducks, geese and pheasants etc. The viruses are negative strand RNA viruses with haemaglutinating activity. Type A, B and C are three antigenically distinct viruses.Type A influenza viruses are found in humans and avian species. Influenza virus from avian sources has been reported to cause fatal influenza in humans in Japan and many Asiatic countries. Influenza virus remains alive for 10 days in dead birds and the virus can infect man and pigs following contact with infected humans, fowls, eggs and raw poultry products. H5N1 viruses with pandemic potential become endemic in some regions of the countries.

Viral replication

Influenza virus A adsorbs to glycoprotein receptors on the cell surface of the avian hosts and enters the cell by receptor mediated endocytosis. The nucleocapsid enters cytoplasm and migrates to the nucleus. Orthomyxoviruses have segmented negative sense RNA genomes. Each segment is transcribed separately by the transcriptase associated with the virus. In short, the virion RNA is transcribed into a positive sense messager RNA depending on the transcriptase carried in the virion. Then, RNA is transcribed from each segement and is translated into single or several proteins. After production and assembly of viral proteins, the RNA influenza virus leaves the cell by budding from the plasma membrane.

Influenza viruses produce mild transient syndromes to 100% morbidity and/or mortality. High morbidity and low mortality is an important feature of avian influenza.

Signs

The important signs are:

1. Decreased activity, low feed consumption, increased broodiness of hens and decreased egg production in chickens. Birds are reported to die en masse.
2. Coughing, sneezing, rales, excesssive lacrimation, huddlings, ruffled feathers, diarrhoea and nervous symptoms in the sick birds
3. Odema of head, face and cyanosis of unfeathered skin are noted in the infected birds.

Age, sex, concurrent infection, strain of virus and environmental factors also influence the symptoms in the sick birds.

Most of the RNA segments encode single proteins in respect of orthomyxoviruses.

Asian influenza virion H5 N1 and another virion H7 have been isolated from bird flu cases in some outbreaks in fowls. The reemergence of this virion has been reported from several Asian countries. The pigs seem to be a mixing vessel where the influenza viral strains exchange gene segments and dangerous viral strains are evolved.

Influenza isolates (surface antigens H7N1 and H7N7) have caused heavy mortality in chickens, turkeys and other species of birds. Influenza virus is infectious for both man and birds but influenza virus types B and C typically infects only man.

Pathology

Gross lesions

These are :

1. Catarrhal, fibrinous, serofibrinous, mucopurulent and caseous lesions are noticed in the sinuses.

2. Oedema of tracheal mucosa with exudate of serous, fibrinous or caseous nature
3. Thickened air sacs and catarrhal or fibrinous peritonitis (particularly egg peritonitis)
4. Presence of catarrhal or fibrinous enteritis in the caeca and or intestines in birds like turkeys. Oviducts of laying birds may contain exudate.
5. Necrotic foci in the liver, spleen, kidneys and lungs in the experimental cases in the chickens. Congested and haemorrhagic wattles and combs in birds affected with some pathogenic viral strains.

Visceral organs may show petechial haemorrhages on their serosol and mucosal surfaces.

Microscopic lesions

The most marked lesions are :

1. Oedema, hyperaemia, haemorrhages and foci of perivasular lymphoid cuffing in some organs like cardiac myocardium, spleen, lungs, brain, wattles, liver and kidneys etc.
2. Presence of parenchymal degeneration and necrosis in spleen, liver and kidneys etc.
3. Focal necrosis, perivascular lymphoid cuffing, glial foci, vascular proliferation and neuronal changes in the brains of infected birds
4. Oedema, hyperaemia, haemorrhagic foci of necrosis are noticed in the spleen, liver, lung, kidneys, intestine and pancreas of experimental chickens infected with influenza virus. Myocarditis with focal areas of necrosis are noticed in experimentally infected chickens. In short, the characteristic lesions of influenza are :
    i). Multiple focal lymphoid necrosis and pancreatic necrosis in infected turkeys

ii). Lesions of focal necrosis in the skelatal muscles, brain, comb and ocular muscles etc. in infected chickens with influenza viruses.

Diagnosis

It is based on the signs, lesions and isolation of the influenza virus. The HI test, virus neutralisation, complement fixation, neuraminidase-inhibition test and ELISA are done to identify and confirm the viral infection.

Treatment /Management

There is no specific treatment of influenza in the affected birds. Amantadine hydrochloride and rimantadine hydrochloride administered in the drinking water reduce the mortality in infected birds. Supportive treatment in view of the respiratory symptoms in the sick birds is advised to protect the birds. Susceptible birds are separated from the infected lot.

Genetic interchange or reassortment between birdflu virues and human virues or mixing of birdflu viruses with human viruses ends in formation of deadly transmissible viruses for humans. Thus, it becomes difficult to control flu in birds and human beings and is considered a very serious disease for birds and human beings.

The important information in relation to control and management of bird flue (avian influenza) are as follows :

1. The strain H5N1 (or a subtype of influenza A) mainly infects the birds but does not affect readily the human beings. On the basis of two proteins, namely, haemagglutinin and neuraminidase, there are 15 subtypes of haemagglutinin (H1 to H15) and nine subtypes of neuraminidase (N1 to N9) respectively.

2. The vaccination programme recommended by FAO is called 'DIVA'(i.e. differentiating infected from vaccinated birds). This technique leads to development of infected birds which

do not reveal clinical symptoms of bird flu but they exist by such vaccination procedure and do not spread this viral disease. Such infected birds or eggs can be used for food purposes. Heterologous vaccines are used to enforce this DIVA technique. In producing effective avian vaccine to control bird flue viral outbreak, there is a need to keep in view the virus H5N1 or its subtypes into consideration.

3. H5 and H7 avian vaccines are available for use of veterinarians in the infected flocks with bird flu.

4. The birds revealing infection with H5N1 are recommended to be culled within 3 Km of the infected poultry form. The surveillance zone spreads over an area of 3 km to 10 km from the poultry farm or flock of infected birds. A period of about 3 months is considered to be safe for trade in poultry and poultry products in the surveillance zone. If infection is not noticed in the vaccinated birds, permission to trade in poultry products is considered. There should be rigorous surveillance and monitoring along with laboratory testing of the infected suspected cases of bird flue to keep the bird free of the avian influenza virus. It has to be kept in mind that vaccination alone cannot get rid of bird flue virus, laboratory testing of suspected cases and culling are also very important steps. A subtype of H5N1 has been noticed with all the genes of avian influenza origin and such mutated viral strain infects both man and birds. Resortment of genes in mammals (say, man) occurs following infections with the common influenza virus and the H5N1 at the same time. Gene mixing between the H5N1 and human influenza virus leads to emergence of new subtype.

5. Heat at 70 degrees centigrade in all parts of eggs or meat of infected birds kills the bird flu virus.

6. Deep frying and boiling (an important Indian style of cooking) kills the bird flu virus (i.e. the H5N1 strain or its mutated subtype).

7. The bird flue virus exists in encrusted forms of faeces or droppings and nasal secretions of the infected birds. Bird flu spreads from birds to birds but does not usually infect human beings. But, the risk of H5N1 (or bird flu) infection to human always remains through emergence of virulent bird flu strains because of mutation or reassortment of genes. Direct contact or close proximity to infected birds can lead to human infection. The reality of one bird flu viral mutant capable of spreading the disease from man to man as a pandemic disease has hitherto not been recorded.

8. Poultry farmers, chicken sellers, handlers and transporters can spread the infection to healthy birds or humans. Use of rubber gloves, eyewears, protective clothings and masks are important precautions against bird flu.

9. Deep burial (i.e. in 6 ft deep trenches between layers of bleach, detergents etc) or even burning of the infected birds is recommended to check its spread.

10. Difficult breathing, high fever, cold, cough, running nose and pain in the muscles of the persons handling or living in close contact with infected lot of birds are important signs of bird flu warranting the need to make immediate contact with medical doctors but the infected birds, showing tremors, diarrhoea, head tilt, staggering and paralysis etc. indicate infection of bird flu in a flock of poultry. Sudden death en masse makes one to suspect bird flu infection but it should be differentiated from other infections of respiratory tract e.g. Ranikhet disease.

25

Favus (Tinea)

Favus is a kind of dermatomycoses involving the skin and its adnexae. *Trichophyton gallinae* causes favus (tinea) in chickens and turkeys. The causative fungi grow in the epithelial cells of the skin and the infection does not extend to the deeper structures. Fungal infections are not frequently noticed in poultry but such infections warrant the need for extensive studies. Fungi like *Geotrichum candidum* and *Trichophyton verricosum* infection have been reported in birds. The fungal growth may cause some thickening of the skin. The periodic acid-shiff (PAS) method is useful to detect fungi in the affected skin. Skin scrappings cleaned with 10 to 40% sodium or potassium hydroxide solution are placed on clean glass slides and examined under the low and high power objectives to detect the fungi.

26

Quail Disease (Ulcerative enteritis)

This disease is caused by *Corynebacterium perdicum*. Contaminated food, water and droppings from the infected birds are sources of infection to healthy birds. It is marked by sudden onset and rapid death of the affected birds. Pigeons and chickens are also susceptible to it.

Signs

These are as under :

1. Affected birds are emaciated and pass white droppings. Mortality in young birds extends up to 100%.
2. Emaciated pectoral muscles. Acute form of quail disease is marked by death within 3 days.

The following are the main lesions :

1. Haemorrhagic duodenitis and punctate haemorrhages in the sick birds
2. Haemorrhagic ulcerative necrotic (diphtheritic) changes in the intestinal walls or caeca of the dead quails. Necrosis in the mucosa of intestine is a marked microscopic lesion.
3. Mottled enlarged liver with yellow or greyish discolouration. Necrotic foci are seen in hepatic parenchyma.
4. Enlarged haemorrhagic spleen in the dead birds

Diagnosis

It is based on the symptoms, lesions, isolation and identification of the organisms from the infected birds. Fluorescent antibody technique and agar gel immunodiffusion test are carried out to confirm the diagnosis of quail disease.

Management /Treatment

Survivors in natural outbreak are carriers of quail disease. Removal of contaminated litter and use of clean litter for each bird is advised to control this disease. There should be no contact between healthy quails and survivors of *Corynabacterium perdicum* infection.Bacitracin (0.005-0.01%) and streptomycin (0.006%) are quite effective in ailing birds.

27

Avian Pseudotuberculosis (AP)

It is a contagious disease of wild and domesticated birds caused by *Yersinia pseudotuberculosis*. The chief features of the disease are as follows :

1. Acute septicaemic infection for a short period
2. Caseous changes (because of chronic inflammation as seen in avian tuberculosis) in liver and lungs etc.

This disease is transmitted through contaminated soil, food or water etc. A state of bacteriaemia develops in the infected birds.

Signs

The main signs are :

1. Sudden death of birds with appearance of diarrhoea and acute septicaemia
2. Weak birds with dull and ruffled feathers
3. A protracted course of disease with weakness, paralysis and emaciation
4. Drooping of wings, constipation and discolouration of skin

Lesions

The important lesions of AP are as under :

1. Enlarged spleen and livers with enteritis. Tubercles-like lesions in different organs
2. Increased amount of fluid in the serous cavities

3. Osteomyelitis or chronic caseous necrotic foci near the growth plates of long bones
4. Degenerative changes (myopathy) in the muscles

Diagnosis

It is based on the symptoms, lesions and isolation of the causative agent i.e. *Y. pseudotuberculosis*.

Treatment/Management

Use or chloramphenicol and streptomycin sulphate (0.6 g and 0.5 g/L) respectively reduces death loss. Treatment with high levels of tetracyclines arrests the disease in flocks. Good management is recommended in poultry farms.

28

Mycoplasma Gallisepticum (MG) Infection (Chronic Respiratory Disease)

This avian infection occurs as a chronic respiratory disease (CRD) of the chickens and infectious sinusitis of turkeys. The main clinical features of the disease are respiratory rales, coughing, nasal discharge and frequent sinusitis in turkeys. This infection develops slowly in birds and has very long course. A disease called air sac disease of poultry is severe air sacculitis due to *M.gallisepticum* along with some concurrent complication of *Eischerichia coli* and respiratory viral agents. The causative agent of CRD is *Mycopolasma gallisepticum* which is very pathogenic for chickens and turkeys. It also occurs in pheasants and quails. Direct contact of the infected birds with healthy flocks and contaminated dusts or water droplets cause transmission of CRD.

Signs

The main clinical signs are :

1. Tracheal rales, gasping, nasal discharge and coughing
2. Reduced feed consumption, loss of body weight and decreased egg production by layers and broilers affected between 4 and 8 weeks of age
3. Foaming eyes with secretion in turkeys due to swelling of paranasal sinuses. Other signs in turkeys are closed eyes, tracheal rales, emaciation, coughing, laboured breathing and drop in egg production.
4. Salpingitis in infected chickens with *M. gallisepticum*

The microscopic changes are :

1. Thickening of the mucous membrane of the affected tissues e.g., respiratory passages due to mononuculear infiltration and hyperplasia of the mucous glands in the affected lungs
2. Pneumonic, granulomatous or lymphofollicular changes in the affected lungs

Diagnosis

The main steps of diagnosis are :

1. Isolation and identification of the causative factor. In complicated cases, *E. coli* and respiratory viruses are found in addition to *M. gallisepticum*.
2. Rapid serum test, tube agglutination test, HI and ELISA tests are useful to diagnose *M. gallisepticum* infection. IB and MG should be differentiated from ND (Newcastle disease) in chickens in flocks with a history of complicated CRD problem.

Management/Treatment

The main steps are :

1. Use of streptomycin, oxytetracyline, chlortetracycline and tylosin etc is recommended in infected flocks of chickens and turkeys.
2. Medicate breeder flocks or their progeny with streptomycin, oxytetracycline, chlortetracyline and tylosin etc. to reduce the rate of MG infection.
4. Egg innoculation is also beneficial in controlling MG infection. Inject lincomycin and spectomycin into the air cells of hatching eggs.
5. Replace infected flocks of chickens and turkeys with flocks free of MG infection. Only replacement flocks free of MG infection are used.

29

Aspergillosis (Brooder Pneumonia)

It is a fungal disease of birds caused by species of the genus *Aspergillus*. The main causative agents of aspergillosis are *A. fumigatus* and *A flavus*. Other involved species in causing brooder pnumonia are *A. terrus and A. glaucus. Aspergillus* spp. is also known to produce aflatoxins but the significance of these toxins in brooder pneumonia is not fully understood. Mortality may reach 50% in the confined flocks of birds. Hyphae of this fungus penetrate the living tissues and form greenish yellow patches on the mucous membranes of air passages. Sick birds die of asphyxiation.

Signs

The main signs are as follows :

1. Dysponea, gasping, noise in trachea and accelerated breathing. Infected birds (5 days of age) show the classical form of aspergillosis.
2. Gurgling and rattling noises in complicated cases of aspergillosis with infectious bronchitis and infectious layngotracheitis
3. Somnolence, inappetence, emaciation, diarrhoea, increased thirst and fever in the infected birds with aspergillosis
4. Other symptoms of *Aspergillus* spp. infection include convulsions, torticollis and lack of equilibirium.

Pathology

The main gross lesions are:

1. Air sacculitis in young chickens and caseous plaques on the

thickened airsac membranes. Fungi and inflammatory exudate are present in the caseous nodules.

2. Presence of visible whitish or greenish grey moldy growth on the caseous lesions. It is worth mentioning that the fungal hyphae also penetrate in the lung parenchyma. Such hyphae are seen on the mucous lining of air passages, in the air sacs in the interior of bones and on the alimentary mucosae.

4. Lungs may reveal diffuse greyish yellow areas in aspergillosis of chicks. Lung nodules and membranous masses of mycelia over the bronchial lining or gelatinous exudate in the infected birds.

5. Yellow circumscribed areas on the brain surface of the infected birds. Caseous coating on lungs or pleura are also noticed.

The main microscopic changes are :

1. Focal accumulation of lymphocytes, macrophages and giant cells in the early lesions of aspergillosis.

2. Granulomatous lesions reveal central areas of necrosis containing heterophils. Such necrotic areas are surrounded by macrophages, giant cells of the foreign body type, lymphocytes and some fibrous tissue. In old lesions (i.e. 8 week postexposure) granulomatous lesions have necrotic centres surrounded by **giant cells of foreign body types** and thick layer of fibrous tissue. In stained sections, the fungi are noticed in the necrotic lesions. Sporulation of fungi or septate branching filaments are noticed in tissue sections of bronchioles and air sacs in the infected birds.

4. The lesions include oedema and infiltration of heterophils, macrophages and cellular debris which are also found in the chambers and retina of the eyes.

5. Thickening and inflammatory changes are noticed in the mucosae of the respiratory tract.

Diagnosis

The main steps are :

1. Isolation and identification of the causative agent
2. Agar gel precipitation and ELISA tests are somewhat useful.
3. Stained sections of the aspergillus nodule with PAS are examined to detect the septate *Aspergillus filaments*.

Management/Treatment

The main steps are :

1. Hatchery sanitation is a very important for controlling *Aspergillus fumigatus* infection. Destroy and burn all the affected chicks.
2. Destroy moldy litter or feed and straw stack etc.
3. Daily cleaning and disinfection of feed and water utensils helps eliminate infection.
4. Maintain proper ventilation in the poultry houses. Provide clean feeds and water to birds.
5. These is no effective therapy against aspergillosis in birds. Prevention is the only reasonable step to control aspergillosis.

30

Thrush (Candidiasis)

It occurs in chickens, pigeons, geese, turkeys, quails and pheasants etc and refers to mycotic infections of the digestive tract. The most frequent cause of moniliasis is *Candida albicans* (i.e a yeast like fungus).

Signs

The main signs are :

1. Poor growth, stunted appearance, listlessness and roughened feathers in the infected birds

Pathology

The main lesions are :

1. The lesions in the crop are thickening of the mucosae with whitish circular raised ulcers. Scales may be noticed on the ulcerative surfaces.
2. Presence of pseudomembranous patches or necrotic material over the mucosae of the crop
3. Ulcerative patches in the mouth and oesophagus. The proventriculus is swollen and its mucosa is haemorrhagic and covered with catarrhal or necrotic exudate.
4. The sections of the crop reveal extensive destruction of stratified epithelium. Walled off ulcers and diphtheritic membranes are the lesions noticed in crop and proventriculus. *C.albicans* is noticed in the stained sections of the lesions.

Diagnosis

It is based on the symptoms, lesions and isolation of *C. albicans* from the lesions.

Treatment/Management

Segregate the affected birds from the healthy ones and apply an antiseptic drug to the oral lesions in the infected birds. 200 mg nystatin/kg diet is effective in eliminating thrush in the ailing turkeys. Nystatin (110 mg/kg ration) gives protection against moniliasis in sick birds. Use of 2000 solution of $CuSO_4$ in drinking water is recommended for infected turkeys.

31

Avian Arizonosis (AA)

It is caused by *Salmonella arizona* (a sub-species of the genus *Salmonella*). Turkeys and chickens are affected. Infected adults are intestinal carriers and intection is transmitted through eggs. The organisms in the droppings of birds penetrate into the shells or eggs.

Signs :

The main signs are:

1. Listlessness, diarrhoea and leg paralysis
2. Other signs include twisted neck, faecal pasting around the vent, and huddling together in poultry shades.

Lesions

These are:

1. Inflammatory, degenerative and necrotic changes in visceral organs
2. Peritonitis, retained yolk sacs, enlarged yellowish mottled liver and discoloured heart are also present.
3. Generalised septicaemia and congested duodenum are noticed.

Diagnosis

It is based on the symptoms, lesions and isolation of the organisms from the liver and heart etc.

Treatment/Management

Sick birds are administered furazolidone and anitibiotics (injectables) like gentamicin and spectinomycin. Disinfection of poultry houses and frequent collections of eggs are also advisable.

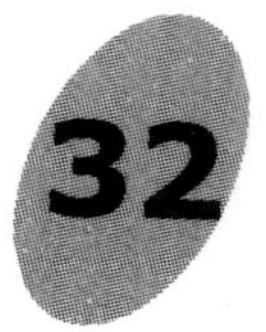

Rupture of the Gastrocnemius Tendon

It leads to lameness in the affected birds like meat type chickens. Birds ailing from bilateral rupture of these tendons sit on their hocks with their toes flexed. A swelling is noticed on the posterior surface of the leg above the hock. Haemorrhages in the lesions with greenish discolouration are noticeable changes. Blood-filled swellings are present on the posterior surface of the legs. Blood in the lesions (i.e. haematomas) may be absorbed and fibrosis encloses the ends of the ruptured tendons. In microscopic sections, synovial hyperplasia and resolving haematomas are important findings. Tenosynovitis due to reovisuses may be implicated in some cases of ruptured gastrocnemius tendon.

Heat Prostration

Birds are very susceptible to high temperatures and abnormal humidity. Birds lack sweat glands and only respiration helps them to overcome the adverse effects of heat. High body temperatures, weakness in birds and death due to respiratory, circulatory and electrolyte imbalances are the main changes in this disorder.

Only spraying the affected birds with water has cooling effects on them. Cooling of the air and adequate drinking of water protects the birds from death.

34

Dehydration

When the birds are unable to drink water or reach the sources of water, they suffer from dehydration. Chicks with no access to water die in 4-5 days. Only fresh water and easy access to it saves the birds from death.

Pathology

The main changes in the dehydrated birds are :

1. Dehydrated and wrinkled skin on the shaft
2. Blue discolouration of the beak
3. Dry and dark breast musculature in the dead birds
4. Dark kidneys with accumulated urates in the ureters
5. Dark blood and loss of body weight

Treatment/Management

There should be easy access to water for all the birds in a flock to prevent the incidence of dehydration. Large or small drinkers must be in proper condition to provide water to birds in flocks. Birds prefer to drink a little amount of water at a time.

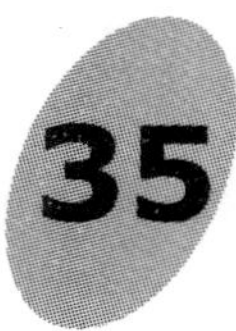

Gangrenous Dermatitis (GD)

It is an infectious disease of chickens from 17 days to 20 weeks of age which is marked by severe necrosis of muscles and subcutaneous tissues. Isolates from the dermal lesions reveal causative factors like *Clostridium perfringens, Cl. septicum* and *Staphylococcus aureus* etc. Natural outbreak of gangrenous dermatitis has been reported in chickens, layers, broilers and breeders etc. Subcutaneous emphysema may also be noticed in such cases and death in GD varies from 1 to 60%. This poultry malady also occurs in India and combined infections of the aforesaid organisms produce severe GD in birds.

Symptoms

Depression, incoordination, inappetence, weakness and ataxia in the affected birds are the main symptoms.

Gross lesions

The lesions are as under :

1. Dark moist areas of skin usually devoid of feathers. Such areas are noticed on the breast, abdomen and legs of sick birds
2. Extensive blood-tinged oedema with or without gas (subcutaneous emphysema)
3. Grey or tan areas in the affected muscles with oedema and gas between muscle bundles
4. Presence of emphysema and serosanguinous fluid in the subcutaneous tissues
5. Discrete white necrotic foci in the liver
6. Light microscopy reveals oedema, emphysema, basophilic

large bacilli, haemorrhages and necorsis in lesions of the affected birds.

Diagonsis

It is based on the symptoms, lesions and isolation of *Clostridia* spp. and staphylococci.

Treatment/Management

Administration of chlortetracyclines, oxytetracyclines and penicillin etc. is advisable. Copper sulphate in water and furoxidine in the feed is also beneficial. Treatment of birds is difficult in avian flock with history of IBD infection (An immunosuppressive disease), avian adenoviruses and reoviruses cases etc. in birds infected with gangrenous dermatitis.

Botulism (Limberneck)

It is an intoxication in the birds caused by an exotoxin of *Clostridium botulinum* type C. Other toxin types e.g. *Cl. botulinum* type D and *Cl. botulinum* type E also induce toxaemic state in birds. Poultry consuming decomposed or rotten vegetable matters, decaying carcasses and contaminated feeds etc. with *Cl.botulinum* suffer from limberneck. Sick birds show difficult breathing due to partial paralysis of the respiratory muscles and dropped wings. Incubation period ranges from 1 to 2 days and mortality may reach 40% in broiler chickens.

Symptoms

The main signs are :

1. Flaccid paralysis of legs, wing, neck and eyes in infected birds
2. Paralytic signs in wings, neck and eyelids. Paralysis of the neck (i.e. limberneck) is a characteristic sign of *Cl. botulinum* infection in the sick birds which are unable to hold up their heads.

In neurotransmission, acetylcholine is released by nerve impulse at the efferent (motor end) plates to trigger a muscular contraction. Type C toxin blocks or inhibits the release of acetylcholine from synaptic vesicles at synaptic clefts or neuromuscular junctions. As a result, acetylcholine (a neurotransmitter) fails to show the response with consequent paralysis of the muscles (e.g. respiratory muscles). The typical symptom of limberneck is shown by the sick birds. In other words, the affected birds rest their beak on the ground or other objects in the poultry shed.

Lesions

There are no marked gross or microscopic lesions in the cases of limberneck as seen in the animals died of tetanus (*Cl. tetani* infection)

Diagnosis

It is based on the symptoms, absence of any marked gross or microscopic lesions and detection of toxins in the serum, crop or gasterointestineal washings from sick birds. Mice injected with *Cl. botulinum* toxins die.

Treatment/Management

Isolate the sick birds and give fresh water and feed to them. Removal and culling of sick birds, disinfection of poultry houses and fly control are recommended to prevent limberneck in birds. Treatment of a large number of sick birds is not an economically advisable step. However, protection of only valuable exotic or valuable birds is worth treatment. Use of antibiotics like pencillin, chlortetracycline and streptomycin etc. is effective in reducing mortality in the sick birds.

37

Coryza (Infectious Coryza)

Coryza is an infectious disease caused by *Haemophilus paragallinarum*. The terms like roup, cold and infectious catarrh also refer to a same disease called coryza which is known to affect chickens and layers. Birds of all ages are susceptible to *H. paragallinarum* infection. Incubation period is a short one which varies from 24 to 48 hrs. Nasal passages and sinuses of birds are infected by this organism. Thus, coryza is an example of an infectious upper respiratory disease of birds. Hypovitaminosis A produces nutritional roup in birds marked by infectious inflammation of upper respiratory tract like pharynx or syrinx etc.

Signs

The main signs are :

1. Nasal discharge, facial oedema and conjunctivitis. Rales are heard in the sick birds following infection of the lower respiratory tract.
2. Decreased consumption of feeds, diarrhoea and fall in egg production are other important signs of coryza.

Coryza may cause high mortality in susceptible birds but is usually marked by low mortality and high morbidity.

Pathology

Gross lesions

Acute inflammatory lesions are noticed in the mucous membranes of the nasal passages and sinuses.

The main lesions are :

1. Catarrhal conjunctivitis and subcutaneous oedema of face

and wattles

2. Catarrhal exudate on the mucous membranes of nasal passages and sinuses
3. Rare occurrence of pneumonia and air sacculitis

Microscopic lesions

These are :

1. Sloughing, disintegration, hyperplasia of the mucosal and glandular epithelium, oedema and hyperaemia in the tunica propria of the mucous membranes are the changes noticed in the nasal cavity, trachea and infraorbital sinuses.
2. In the cases of catarrhal bronchopneumonia, heterophils and cell debris in the lumens of secondary and tertiary bronchi, hyperplasia and swelling in the epithellum of the air capillary are noteworthy changes.
3. Catarrhal inflammatory changes in the air sacs is marked by infiltration of heterophils.
4. Mucosae of the nasal cavity reveals pronounced infiltration of mast cells.

Diagnosis

It is based on the signs, lesions and isolation of *H. paragallinarum* from the lesions of coryza. Serological tests like plate or tube agglutination, complement fixation, indirect HA, direct fluorescent antibody test are also performed to confirm its diagnosis.

Treatment/Management

Sulfonamides and antibiotics are used to treat the sick birds infected with coryza. Drugs in combination eg. sulfachloropyrazine-sulpadimidine and chlortetracycline-sulfadimethoxine etc. are also quite effective to check mortality and morbidity in the ailing birds.

Recovered birds or chronic cases of IC are carriers. And as such, it is better to replace old birds with fresh day-old chicks. Depopulation of the infected or recovered birds is quite advisable to control incidence of coryza. Houses and equipments should be disinfected to avoid infection of the healthy baby chicks.

The coryza is a bacterial disease caused by *Haemophilus paragallinarum* with high morbidity and as such, treatment or step on time is very much warranted for. After confirmation of the disease by culture examination, the following drugs are used for treating coryza:

(i) Sulphamezathine 16% solution @ 30 ml in 4 litres of water can be given for 3 to 6 days.

(ii) Avisol 4 ml in 4 litres of water can be used for 4 to 6 days.

(iii) Other drugs like diadine, sulmet and vetydine can be used. Supportive treatment in the form of Vitalblend or Vimeral syrup can be given.

Sulpha drugs are very effective in treating infections like coryza with good response from sick birds. Recovered birds act as sources of infection. Only day-old clean chicks should be obtained for replacement purpose. Vaccines have been tried to eradicate the disease. The flocks which have experience of the disease, should be depopulated. It is a known fact that all recovered birds are resevoirs of this infection. It is better to market the birds and premises should be disinfected before addition of new chicks i.e clean birds. Streptomycin and the tetracyclines can be given to the sick birds for a period up to 7 days at the following rates:

Streptomycin - 2.5 mg in chicken 1/m daily for 3 to 6 days.

Tetracyclines - 20-50 mg per kg body weight in water for 3 to 5 days.

38

Paratyphoid (PT) Infections

Paratyphoid infections in poultry, chickens, turkeys and pigeons etc. are caused by hundreds of paratyphoid serotypes. Young birds and chicks during the first two weeks after hatching are frequently affected. Mortality rates among young birds may reach over 80% or higher in some outbreaks. Some important organisms of PT groups are *S. bareilly, S. typhi and S. dublin* etc. Salmonellae are isolated from the faeces of birds and these organisms contain endotoxins associated with the somatic portion of the organisms. Infections in poultry are important sources of food poisoning in humans. Direct ovarian transmission of PT infections is noticed in turkeys. *S typhimurium* penetrate into the egg shell and grow within the eggs. Contaminated poultry feeds and crates and incubators spread infection to other healthy chickens. PT infections produce acute septicaemia in the infected birds.

Signs

The important signs of PT infections are as follows :

1. Somnolence with lowered head, restlessness, depression in young birds with closed eyes and wings drooping with ruffled feathers are noticed.
2. Marked anorexia, increased water consumption, profuse watery excreta with pasting of vent and tendency of huddling near the source of heat and greenish diarrhoea are other important signs in young birds.
3. Inappetence, increased water consumption, diarrhoea, dehydration, droopy wings are noticed in adult birds.

Gross and microscopic lesions

These are as follows :

A. Lesions in young birds.

1. Emaciation, dehydration, coagulated yolks, congested liver and spleen with petechiae or pinpoint necrotic foci
2. Pericarditis with adhesions, congested kidneys, haemorrhagic enteritis (particularly involving duodenum)
3. Some other lesions are like necrotic foci in liver and heart and airsac involvement etc
4. Heterophilic leucopenia with increase in percentage of lymphocytes
5. Duck infected with salmonellae show necrotic foci in the liver, cheesy plugs in caeca, impaction of the cloaca and blanching of kidneys etc.
6. Swollen eyelids, arthritis, subcutaneous swellings and green fibrinous deposits in the oral cavity are the lesions reported in PT infection in pigeons.

B. Lesions in adult birds

Swollen organs like liver, spleen and kidneys and haemorrhagic or necrotic enteritis are the lesions in the adult birds. Other lesions like pericarditis, peritonitis, necrotic or hyperplastic lesions in the oviduct and suppurative and necrotic lesions in the ovaries are noticed in acutely infected birds. Decrease in packed cell volume, haemoglobin and total red cell count, increased sedimentation and total leucocyte count are some haematological findings in the infected birds.

Diagnosis

It is based on the clinical findings, postmortem lesions, isolation and identification of the causative agents and macroscopic tube agglutination test and rapid whole blood test etc. Complement fixation and ELISA are also performed to confirm it.

Treatment/Management

Furazolidone, injectable gentamycin and spectinomycin are quite effective in paratyphoid infections in birds like chickens and turkeys. Recovered birds remain as carriers of *Salmonella* spp. like *S. typhimurium*. Contamination of chickens and breeder hatchery in poultry farms should be avoided. Infected flocks are not used as source of hatching eggs. It is better to dispose of the infected flocks in proper manner (by burning or by deep burial between two layers of lime or any detergent). Eggs of clean flocks are segregated from the eggs of infected flocks. Litter is sprayed with 4 or 6% solutions of formalin with intermittent litter turnover. Inactivated antigens i.e. a formalised broth culture vaccine from a strain of *S. stanley* has been effective in controlling salmonellosis.

39 Mycotoxicosis

Hot and humid climate and lack of storage and handling facilities lead to formation of mycotoxins in certain feed stuffs like groundnut cake and maize etc. Aflatoxin, ochratoxin, fusariotoxin, trichothecenes (like T_2 toxin), rubratoxin, tremorgenic toxin and stachybotrytoxin are some important mycotoxins. The disease processes caused by these toxins in the bodies of animals and birds etc are called mycotoxicoses.Some details of mycotoxicoses in the poultry are given in table 15.

Ducks and chickens ingesting feeds contaminated by *Aspergillus flavus* and *Aspergillus parasiticus* etc develop aflatoxicosis. Poultry susceptibility to aflatoxin is variable but ducks are very susceptible to it. Neoplasms are noticed in the ducks suffering from chronic aflatoxicosis and these growths may be present in the organs like liver, gall bladder and pancreas etc. Aflatoxin B is a highly potent hepatocarcinogen. The main signs in ducks are in appetence, reduced growth, abnormal crying, ataxia, convulsions and opisthotonus. Enlarged and pale livers in acute cases and shrunken firm, nodular growths and distended gall bladder in chronic aflatoxocosis are some gross lesions. Vacuoles, degenerated nuclei, islands of liver cells, regenerated hepatocytes and proliferated bile ducts are important histologic lesions. The main hepatic lesions in subacute aflatoxicosis in chickens are white foci, multiple haemorrhages and pale yellow discolouration of the liver parenchyma. Fatty vacuolation, regenerated hepatocytes and proliferated bile ducts are the lesions noticed in the affected chickens with aflatoxicosis.

Table 15. Different mycotoxicoses of poultry caused by toxic fungal metabolites

Toxins	Diseases caused	Signs	Lesions	Remarks
1. Aflatoxins (produced by *Aspergillus flavus*, A. *parasiticus and Penicillium puberulum* present in any feed or grain for birds and animals. B1, B2, G1 and G2 are some types of aflatoxins designated on the basis of blue and green colour reactions to fluorescent light.	Aflatoxicosis types are acute subacute and chronic.	1. Inappetence, reduced growth and lameness. 2. Convulsions and opisthotonus before death.	1. Livers and kidneys are enlarged and pale. Dark (congested) livers 2. Haemorrhages on kidneys and pancreas etc. 3. Shrunken, firm, nodular liver with distended gall bladder 4. Hepatocytes swollen, enlarged vacuolated with degenerated nuclear material. 5. Bilduct proliferation, extensive fibrosis and islands of hepatocytes. 6. Increase in collagen, reticulum fibres and hyperplasia of reticulon-dothelial cells in chronic or aflatoxicosis of longer duration.	1. Aflatoxin B1 is a hepato carcinogen

Toxins	Diseases caused	Signs	Lesions	Remarks
2. Ochratoxins produced by *Penicillum viridicatum Aspergillus ochraceous*. Toxins present in grains and feed stuffs, toxins are Ochratoxins (A,B, and C.)	Ochratoxicosis	1. Growth rate, and feed consumption affected 2. Diarrhoea with high urate content. 3. Sexual maturity delayed.	1. Pale and swollen kidneys with urates on heart, kidneys, liver and spleen etc. 2. Cytoplasmic vacuolation and focal necrosis of hepatocytes with some fibrosis. 3. Acute tublar nephrosis with proteinaceous and urate casts, interstitium infiltrated with inflammatory cells and glomerular basement membrane thickened. E.M. studies of normal epthelium of the proximal convoluted tubules reveal ring forms of mitochondria, intranuclear and cytoplasmic liquid droplets and electron dense round bodies in smooth endopolasmic reticulum.	1. Immunosuppressive effects 2. Phagocytic activity impaired

Toxins	Diseases caused	Signs	Lesions	Remarks
3. Trichothecenes produced by *Fusarium, Myrothecium* and *Trichothecium* etc. T-2 toxin, diacetoxyscir penol and nivalenol present in feed stuffs like corn and oats etc. T-2 toxin, neosolaniol,verruc arol, fusarenon-X and crotocol are trichothecenes identified in feeds.	Trichothecene mycotoxicosis	1. Depression, recum-bency, feed refusal and cyanotic comb and wattles 2. Reduction in feed intake and thin-shelled eggs.	1. Yellow tan friable livers, swollen kidneys with urates in ureters. Yellow exudate and focal ulceration of crop mucosa. 2. Exudate with underlying ulcers near salivary duct opening on the palate, tongue and buccal floor. Necrosis and ulceration in the mucosa 3. Necrosis of lymphoid and haematopoietic tissues. 4. Haemorrhages and bile duct proliferation in the livers 5. Pale and yellow bone marrow. 6. Gizzard lining thickened, fissured and ulcerated.	

Note : The genus *Fusarium* produces mycotoxins harmful to poultry and some of these toxins are like trichothecenes, T-2 toxin, diacetoxyscirpenol (DAS), deoxynivalenol (DON, vomitoxin). Fusarochromanone is present in water soluble extracts of fusarial species. These are the following:

Toxins	Diseases caused	Signs	Lesions	Remarks
A. Deoxynivalenol (DON)/vomitoxin by *Fusarium roseum*	DON mycotoxicosis	1. Lower feed consumption 2. Higher mortality 3. Diarrhoea 4. Dicreased haemoglobin values	1. Diffuse subcutaneous haemorrhages 2. Visceral gout and ecchymosis in the viscera 3. Mild erosion in the gizzard	
B. Zearalenone present in feed contaminated with *Gibberella zeae* (*Fusarium graminearum*) etc.	Zeralenone mycotoxicosis	1. Peak egg production decreased 2. High mortality in broiler breeders	1. Oviduct distended with fibrinous material 2. Caseous cysts in peritoneum and ascites 3. Increase in weight of bursa of Fabricius. 4. Egg shell thickness reduced and spermatogenesis inhibited by *Fusarium* spp. in geese.	

Toxins	Diseases caused	Signs	Lesions	Remarks
C. Fusarochromanone. This toxin is present in feeds contaminated with *Fusarium roseum* or in cultures of *Fusarium* or in cultures of *Aspergillus niger*, *A.flavus*, *Fusarium moniliforme*	Fusarochromanone mycotoxicosis	Unmineralised avascular zone in the growth plate with crenated and eosinophlic chondrocytes	1. Tibial dyschrondroplasia and (defect in endochondral ossitication is noticed in chickens, turkeys and ducks. 2. Lower density of chondroblasts in stained sections of hypertrophic cartilage.	
4. Ergot alkaloids. These mycotoxins are present in sclerotium of *Claviceps* spp growing in cereal grains e.g., rye and wheat etc.	Ergotism	1. Hypertension leading to cardiac enlargement	1. Combs and wattles atrophied and disfigured 2. Vesicles develop on legs shanks, tops and sides of toes and rupture to form ulcers 3. Vasoconstrucive injuries produced. Liver and kidneys are congested.	

Birds injesting ergot alkaloids suffer from ergotism and show vasoconstrictive effects of ergot. Vesicles appear on the comb, wattles, eyelids, shanks, tops and sides of the toes etc. Crusts develop owing to rupture of these vesicles and atrophied and disfigured combs are seen in the ailing birds. Mycotoxins are formed within the sclerotium when fungi like *Claviceps* attack cereal grains like wheat and rye etc.

Diagnosis

Retarded growth, anaemia, nephrosis, and lesions etc. are of no specific value for the sake of diagnosis. History of change of feed lot or any of its ingredients, no effect of antibiotic treatment and vitamin supplementation, retardation in body growth and occurrence of the disease in the flock during or after rainy season (favouring growth of fungi in the feed stuff) indicate the possibility of mycotoxiosis in birds. A sample of the feed (at least 4 kg) is preserved at 4°c for analysis of the feed for detection of toxins in the infected feed lot.

Other laboratory tests include isolation and indentification of the mycotoxin in the infected food grains, biological test involving injection of the extract of the feed in the susceptible hosts e.g. chick embryo or ducklings. Serological tests are of no use for non-antigenic mycotoxins.

Management/Treatment

There should be proper ventilation in the feed store and the moisture content of the stuff is preferred at 10% level. Spray the floor with 0.5 to 1% of solution of pentachlorophenol in the poultry house.

The quantity of vitamin and protein is increased in the feed stuff to check severity of toxicosis. Aureomycin in the feed stuff is fed to the poultry to control mycotoxicosis in birds. Gentian violet in the diet inhibits growth of fungi and bacteria like staphylococci and *Clostridium* spp. 25g of gentian violet in one ton of feed is recommended in poultry feed to check fungal growth. The growth of *A.flavus, A fumigatus, Fussarium oxysporum, F. moniliforme* and *Candida* spp. is inhibited by gential violet. Several organic acids like propiorates, acetates and fumarates and aluminesilicates are reported to bind mycotoxins like aflatoxin, vomitoxin, ocharatoxin, zearalenone and fusarium toxins. And as such, these substances are added to the feed having moisture content between 14 and 15% at the rate of 2.5 kg per tonne. Addition of hydrated sodium, calcium, aluminosilicate (HSCAS) at a level of 0.5% absorbs aflatoxins in feeds and provides protection against aflatoxicosis. Removal of toxic feed with mycotoxin free feed stuffs is a most important step in prevention of mycotoxicosis in poultry flock. On-site screening tests should be carried out to detect mycotoxins like aflatoxin, T-2 toxin, ochratoxin and zearalenone in the feeds under a quality control programme.

40

Miscellaneous Conditions/Diseases

Cannibalism

The term cannibalism refers to a habit or a vice sometimes shown by poultry of picking one another's feathers, toes, vents, combs and other parts of the body. Its main sign is feather-picking. The blood escapes from the injured tissues (skin etc.) and other birds are attracted towards oozing blood from the skin. Moreover, damage is caused to such birds by fellow birds by pecking or picking.

The main causes are :

1. Close confinement or overcrowded housing conditions
2. Idleness
3. Dietary (nutritional and mineral deficiencies i.e. diet deficient in protein or essential amino acids). Insufficient feeding can also produce this condition in the birds.
4. Presence of itch mites at the base of the feather i.e. irritation by external parasites. Feather-pulling, vent-picking and head or tail-picking are noticed in the affected birds.

Types of cannibalism

These are as follows:

1. Vent-picking
2. Feather-pulling
3. Toe-picking
4. Head-picking
5. Head and tail-picking

Vent-picking

There is a picking of the vent or the region of the abdomen. It is seen in pullet flocks in high production. Prolapses and tearing of the tissues by passage of very large eggs cause blood to escape and the birds are attracted to eat the blood. Such birds develop habit of vent-picking. Anaemia and blood on the tail feathers, the back of legs and injured vent are important findings in dead birds.

Feather-pulling

It is seen in flocks kept in close confinement. The birds have lack of sufficient exercise. Nutritional and mineral deficiencies and irritatrion by lice and mites are contributing factors.

Toe-picking

It is seen in domestic chicks. The vice arises from hunger and inadequate feeder space. When the chicks do not get feed, they pick at their own or others' feet.

Head-picking

Injuries to head, comb and wattles leads to head picking in the birds. The affected birds show black and necrotic ear lobes and blackening around eyes and wattles due to subcutaneous haemorrhages. This vice is seen even in the debeaked birds.

Wing and tail-picking

Feather-pulling and external injuries give rise to this vice in the birds. The birds pick at the feather follicles and drink the oozing blood and start picking at some lesions on the foot and other parts of the body.

Treatment/Management

In order to control cannibalism in birds, over-crowding should be avoided and dietary deficiency of protein, hard grains and salt etc. should be corrected. Debeaking can also be done to check feather-picking.

Subcutaneous emphysema (windpuff)

It arises from some defects or injuries in the respiratory tract which permits accumulation of air beneath the skin. Rough handling, feather-picking, cannibalism, puncturing the skin, fracture of pneumotic bones like humerus and sternum and caponizing may also cause wind puff in birds.

Salt poisoning (Sodium chloride poisoning) in birds

There is a great susceptibility to salt poisoning in chickens, turkeys, ducks and pigeons. It can be acute or chronic. Acute cases results from high intake of salt in the form of brine or fish brine etc. Chronic salt poisonning results from intake of well or pound water. Excess of salt in the feed can cause chronic poisoning. Sodium chloride solution (even physiologic salt solution) can be fatal for baby chicks consuming it for some days. Concentration of salt (about 3 .5%) are toxic for birds. In short, sodium chloride (0.5% or above) in water is toxic for chickens.

Signs

Loss of appetite, somnolence, dyspnoea, thirst, opisthotonus, diarrhoea, convulsions and inability to stand are important signs of salt poisonings. There is an increased intake of water in birds eating feeds rich in salt.

PATHOLOGY

The important pathological changes are ascites, anasarca, hydropericardium, oedema and congestion of lungs. There may be enteritis with oedematous changes. Nephritis, subcutaneous oedema and myocardial haemorrhages can also be found. Visceral gout and impacted ureters are noticed.

TREATMENT

A balanced poultry feed containing 0.37-0.5% sodium chloride should be given to the birds and there should be immediate change of the old feed lot which has led to appearance of such symptoms and lesions of salt poisoning.

Ascites/oedema

In this disease, noninflammatory fluid accumulates in the body cavities or interstitial tissues of organs. Such fluid may be blood-stained or clear yellow in colour and accumulates in the peritoneal, pericardial and thoracic or peritoneal spaces. Ascites secondary to right ventriculr failure (ARVF) is noticed in bröiler chickens and meat-type ducklings.

Causes

These are as follows :

(i) Vascular damage causing leakage of protein rich fluid from the capillaries. Such damage to the blood vessels can be caused by toxic substances.

(ii) Increased vascular hydraulic pressure. Right ventricular (RVF) failure occurs in chickens from pulmonary hypertension which may be secondary to hypervolaemia due to increased dietary sodium (sodium toxicosis). Such hypertension may be primary or spontaneous in nature. Right ventricle undergoes hypertrophy followed by dilatation. The left ventricular wall may be thickened as a secondary condition to RVF.

(iii) Prevention of resorption of tissue fluid due to portal hypertension following right AV valvular insufficiency

(iv) Increased tissue vascular oncotic pressure (usually colloidal)

(v) Decreased vascular oncotic pressure

(vi) Blockage of lymph drainage

(vii) Respiratory aspergillosis.

(viii) Low level of dietary sodium.

(ix) Patent foramen ovale.

(x) Cold and hypoxia causing oedema.

(xi) Even liver congestion leads to oedematous state in the body.

It can also arise from hepatic fibrosis or amyloidosis.

(xii) Virus-like particles detected between the myocardial fibres and in the livers, lungs and kidneys of the affected birds with ARVF.

PATHOLOGY

The main lesions are :

(1) Pale head, shrunken comb and loss of bright white sheen of feathers

(2) Red abdominal skin and congestion of peripheral vessels

(3) Distension of abdomen with fluid. Lungs are oedematous, hyperaemic and haemorrhagic.

(4) Clear yellow fluid or clots of fibrin in the abdomen

(5) Swollen and congested liver. Sinusoidal dilation, capsular thickening and foci of lymphocytes and heterophils are seen in the affected livers.

(6) Presence of mild or severe hydropericardium

(7) Right ventricular dilation or hypertrophy of the right ventricular wall due to pulmonary hypertension. Right auricle and venacavae may be distended with blood.

(8) Occurrence of such condition along with infectious bursal disease (Gumboro disease). The bursa can be found severly enlarged and oedematous with red or pink colouration. It may contain pink-stained mucoid material.

(9) Thining of left ventricular wall. Lungs may be congested and oedematous.

Control

(1) Proper temperature, humidity and air movement should be maintained. The birds should be protected from chills or cold.

(2) The sodium level in the feed is to be kept at 200 ppm. There should be routine analysis of the poultry feeds for sodium or Nacl. In short, common salt (Nacl) is to be kept at level of 0.37-0.5% in the poultry feeds.

(3) Birds are not to be given water containing 500 ppm. of sodium.

(4) Mouldy feeds should not be given to birds to protect them from aspergillosis or aflatoxicosis.

Egg Drop Syndrome (EDS)

This disease is caused by an adenovirus (EDS 76) and marked by a great loss of egg production. Sporadic outbreaks of EDS can occur due to infection of healthy fowls from infected wild or domestic water fowls through direct or indirect contacts.

There is a loss of colour in the pigmented eggs.The eggs are thin shelled, soft-shelled or even shell less. The thin-shelled eggs have a rough sandpaper-like appearance (i.e. the shell has a granular roughing). Egg production can drop to 40%. The affected birds look healthy. In experimentally-affected birds 7-20 days post-infection, there is a marked replication of the virus in the pouch shell gland. Such replication of the virus can be found to lesser extent in other parts of the oviduct. Inflammatory changes are noticed in the pouch shell gland. Abnormal changes are noticed in the pouch shell gland with laying of abnormally shelled eggs. In short, eggs show a loss of shell strength and pigmentation.

PATHOLOGY

Inactive ovaries and atrophied oviducts are found in the affected birds. In experimental cases in fowls, oedema of uterine folds and presence of exudate in the pouch shell are important lesions. Splenomegaly and eggs in the various stages of development can be found.

Diagnosis

It is based on the symptoms and lesions. Attempts are made to isolate and identify the causative factors and cytopathic effects are noticed in the infected tissues. The HI, ELISA, SN and FA tests are quite sensitive tests to diagnose it. HI test is a test of choice to diagnose it.

TREATMENT

The treatment is not successful. Vitamins, increase in calcium or protein in ration do not produce beneficial effects in the infected birds. Vaccination is done to control endemic EDS.The vaccine is injected intramuscularly in the birds between 14 and 18 weeks of age. Chlorinated water can be given to sick birds. Even AE vaccine in water given at the age of 8 to 16 weeks protects the birds against EDS.

Pesticide poisoning

Organochlorines or organochlorides (D.D.T., D.D.E.) and toxaphene are pesticides causing poisoning in birds. The important effects are decreased egg production, thinning of the egg shells, osteomalacia, fall in hatchability, fatty changes in the liver, petechiae under the gizzard epithelium and renal degeneration (nephrosis). Pesticides are estimated in the feeds for diagnosis. Change of poultry feeds in the affected flocks is the immediate step to be undertaken. Organophosphates (e.g. dichlorvos, malathion and parathion) produce incordination, staggering, paralysis, dyspnoea and convulsions (neurotoxicity) following ingestion and absorption of such insecticides. Birds died of poisons or ingestion of pesticides are unfit for human or animal consumption and should be incineratad or buried in deep trenches in a proper manner.

Insecticides like organophophates, organochlorides and carbamates cause toxicity in birds like poultry and water fowls etc. following the ingestion of such substances. The main signs in the affected birds are as follow

Insecticides/Pesticides	Signs and lesions
1. Organochlorides	a) Convulsions (tremors), ataxia, salivation, depression and death b) Diarrhoea, decreased egg production, drop in hatchability, embryo moratlity, depigmentation of eggs, chalky eggs, egg shell thinning and congestion and haemorrhages are noticed in the affected birds

Insecticides/Pesticides	Signs and lesions
2. Organophosphates and Carbamates High susceptibility of chickens and birds to these products. Acetylcholinesterase is inhibited by these insecticides and accumulation of acetylcholine causes over-stimulation of parasympathetic nerves and muscles with fatal consequences	a) Convulsions (tremors), incordination, dullness, depression, lacrimation, dyspnoea and paralysis are some signs of poisonings b) Presence of congestion and haemorrhages in the cardiac muscles, on serosal surface and on intestinal mucosa in the dead birds

APPENDIX

Contents of the appendix

(a) Antibiotics and other drugs used in the treatment of poultry diseases

(b) Stains and reagents commonly used in the laboratories

(c) Faecal examination

(d) Poultry feed formulae

(e) Some common preservatives

(f) Some useful insecticides

(g) Examination of ectoparasites and fungi

(h) Avian autopsy technique (Rubarth, 1964)

(i) Red and white blood cells

(j) Rapid method for staining spirochaetes

(k) Normal range of blood values of poultry

(l) Diseases of zoo,wild and laboratory animals

A. TABLE 16. ANTIBIOTICS AND OTHER DRUGS USED IN THE TREATMENT OF POULTRY DISEASES

Sl. No.	Compounds	Indications	Methods of application	Dose rates	Duration Days)
1.	Ampicillin	Salmonellosis, *E.coli* and staphylococcosis	Water	12.5 mg/kg	4-5
2.	Chlortetracycline	Colibacillosis, salmonellosis respiratory disease complex, necrotic enteritis and stress	Water	25g/185-L	4-5
3.	Mythromycin	Mycoplasma infection (CRD), streptococcosis, coryza and necrotic dermatitis	Water	25g/225-L	4-5
4.	Furaltadone	Colibacillosis, salmonellosis respiratory disease complex and stress	Water	500g/800-L	5-7
5.	Furazolidone 20%	Colibacillosis, salmonellosis CRD complex and stress	Feed	2 kg/t	5-7
6.	Lincospectin	CRD	Water	37.5mg/bird	1 day
7.	Oxytetracycline	Colibacillosis, salmonellosis , necrotic enteritis, respiratory disease complex and stress	Water/Feed	25g/185-L/220g/t	4-5 5-7
8.	Trimethoprim	*E. coli* infection, *Haemophilus* sp. infection, pasteurellosis and salmonellosis	Water	30 mg/kg bwt.	3-5
9.	Enrofloxacin	Mycoplasmosis, staphylococcosis and *E. Coli* infection	Water	2-5 mg/kg bwt	3-5
10.	Penicillin	Spirochaetosis and necrotic enteritis	Feed	220g/t	5-7

Sl. No.	Compounds	Indications	Methods of application	Dose rates	Duration Days)
11.	Sulmet 12.5%solution	Coryza, cholera and coccidioisis	Water	30g/L	2 days followed by 1/2 dose for 4 days
12	Sulphaqinoxa-line7%	Coccidiosis and cholera	Water	30g/5L	3 days and off1 and repeat
13	Tylan sol	Mycoplasma infection	Water	35-110mg/bird	1-2
14.	Tylan inj.	Do	Subcutaneous injection	0.5-2cc/bird	Once
15.	Amprol plus sol	Coccidiosis	Water	60ml/20L	5-7
16.	Levamisole	All intestinal species (i.e. Gut round worms)	Water	18 to 50 mg/kg b.wt.	24 hours
17.	Phenothiazine	All species of intestinal parasites	Water	0.5-1g/bird	6-7 hours
18	Piperazine	*Ascardia* spp.	Water	145g/450kg	3-4 hours
19	Mebendazole	Gut round worms, tapeworms and Syngamus	Water	10 mg/kg b.wt	3 days
20.	Sulphametazine	Coccidiosis	Water	0.1%, 05%	2 days 4 days
21.	Amprolium	Coccidiosis	Water	0.012-0.024% 3-5 days;0.006%	1 to 2 weeks
22.	Sulfadimethoxine	Coccidiosis	Water	0.05%:	6 days
23.	Aftox (a combination of co-pper sulphate, propionic acid and glacial acetic acid)	Mycotoxicosis(aflatoxicosis, aspergillosis and candidiasis), haemorrhagic enteritis, *E. coli*, salmonellosis, Ranikhet disease, infectious bursal disease	Water	1-2ml/L (curative) 2ml/L (prophylactic)	4-6 days only two hours on first day and then repeat after 10th/20th and 30th day.

Sl. No.	Compounds	Indications	Methods of application	Dose rates	Duration Days)
24.	Cotrim (cotrim-oxazole)	Bacillary diarrhoea, coccidiosis, colibacillosis, IC, CRD, and infections of urogenital and gastero intestinal tracts.	Water	2 gm/L	3-5d ays
25.	Ciproxin (Cipro-floxacin 10% w/w)	Mycoplasmosis, bacterial and viral infections	Water	Chicks-1gm/2L Broilers-1gm/L	5-7 days
26.	Roxicin forte (Roxithromycin 10% w/w)	CRD, fowl cholera, *E.Coli,* salmonellosis and aspergillosis	Water	Chicks 1g/4L Broilers and layers 1gm/2L In serious cases 1 gm/L	
27.	Ionophorous antibiotics (lasalocid)	Coccidiosis	Feed	75-125 ppm	5-7 days
28.	Quinolones(Decoquinate)	do	Feed	30 ppm	do
29.	Pyridones	do	Feed	125-250 ppm	do
30.	Carbanilide(Nicarbazin)	do	Feed	125 ppm	do

Note

t= tonne

l= litre

b.wt= body weight

B. STAINS AND REAGENTS COMMONLY USED IN LABORATORIES

These are as follows:

(1) Leishman's stain

(2) Giemsa's stain

(3) 1% Crystal violet solution

(4) Ziehl Neelsen's carbol solution

(5) 1% methylene blue solution

(6) Gram's iodine

(7) 2-3% Acid alcohol

(8) 95% Absolute alcohol

Films or smears of blood and exudate etc. are made on clean glass slides to detect bacteria and protozoa etc. Thin films are usually prepared but thick films are made in some diseases (for example, anthrax). Details of the stains and procedures followed are given below :

(a) Leishman's stain

It is prepared by dissolving 0.15g Leishman's powder in 100cc pure acetone-free methyl alcohol. It is quite good for differential count as well as for staining bacteria and protozoa in films and sections.

Buffer $Na_2\ HPo_4\ 12H_2O$(sodium phosphate)	35.61 g to litre
$NaH_2\ Po_4\ 2H_2O$(sodium dihydrogen phosphate)	27.61 g to litre

Autoclave it at 15 lbs (pressure) per sq. inch for 30 minutes. And keep it in cold stores.

Procedure

(1) Pour the Leishman's stain on the unfixed smear or blood films and leave it to act for 1 minute. Methyl alcohol in the

stain fixes the smears on the glass slides.

(2) Add double the volume of freshly-prepared distilled water or buffer solution (i.e 1 part of the stain and 2 parts of distilled water at neutral pH) on to the slide and mix the stain and buffer with a Pasteur pipette by sucking it up in the pipette and expelling it out on the slide.

(3) Allow the diluted stain to act for 5 to 10 minutes depending upon the quality of the Leishman's stain.

(4) Examine under the oil immersion objective after taking one or two drops of cedar wood oil or even liquid paraffin. Interacorpuscular parasites (e.g. *Babesia spp.*) are usually seen at the margins and termination of the films in mammals. Leucocytozoon in peripheral blood films of chickens is stained with brilliant cresyl blue. Plasmodium is stained in the red cells by any Romanowsky stain. The initial stage of the merozoites occurs in the ring forms in the red cells and a vacuole is noticed in the parasites. Haemoproteus infects red cells of pigeons. Trypanosomes also infects domestic and wild birds.

(b) Giemsa's stain

It is prepared by dissolving 3.8 g of Giemsa's stain in 250 ml pure methyl alcohol (acetone free) by shaking for 15 minutes and then it is added to 250 ml of glycerine. The mixture is shaken for 10 minutes. Filter the stain and discard the residue. It keeps very well. Good for bacteria and protozoa in the smears. It can be used for staining pasteurella, chlamydial inclusion bodies, haemophilus and spirochaetes.

Procedure

(1) Fix smear or blood film with methly alcohol for 2 minutes.

(2) Stain with dilute Giemsa's stain (2 drops of stock Giemsa's solution in 1 ml of buffer, pH6.8) or freshly prepared distilled water for 30 minutes to one hour in view of the quality of

the stain.

(3) Wash with the same buffer solution or distilled water.

(4) Dry in the air, add a drop of cedar wood oil on the smear and examine under oil immersion objective.

(c) Gram's stain

Solutions required :

(1) 1% Crystal violet solution

(2) Gram's iodine or Lugol's iodine solution

Lugol's iodine solution

Iodine	1g
Potassium iodide	2 g
Water	300 ml.

(3) Dilute carbol fuchsin

It is prepared by mixing 1 part of Ziehl Neelsen stain with nine parts of distilled water.

(4) 95% absolute alcohol

Procedure

(i) Smears from tissues or exudate are made, dried in the air and fixed by heat.

(ii) Stain smears for 1 minute with 1% crystal violet solution.

(iii) Wash the smears in tap water for about 2 seconds and add iodine solution on to the smears and allow it to act for 1 to 2 minutes.

(iv) Wash in tap water and decolourise the smears with 95% absolute alcohol for 30 seconds and wash again the smears in tap water.

(v) Counterstain the smears with dilute carbol fuchsin for 10 seconds.

(vi) Wash in tap water, dry and examine under oil immersion objective.

Note: Gram positive bacteria stain blue or violet but the gram negative organisms stain red or pink.

Ziehl-Neelsen's stain

Good for acid fast bacteria or spores in the films or sections.

Solutions required are :

(1) Ziehl-Neelsen's stain

It is prepared by dissolving one gram basic fuchsin in 10 ml absolute alcohol and 100ml of an aqueous solution of carbolic acid(1to 20) is then added to it. The dye is at first dissolved in the absolute alcohol and, then, the die in alcohol is added to the phenol solution in the distilled water.

(2) 3% acid alcohol

Hydrochloric acid	3 ml
70% alcohol	97 ml.

(3) 1% aqueous solution of methylene blue

Procedure

(1) Stain the dried and fixed smear with Z.N. stain. Smear is flooded with the stain and is heated until the steam rises and the hot stain is allowed to act for 2 minutes. Heat can be applied at intervals to keep it hot.

(2) Wash with water.

(3) Decolourise the smears, until the smears are faintly pink.

(4) Wash the smears in tap water and counter stain with 1% methylene blue for 10 to 20 seconds.

(5) Wash, dry and examine it under oil immersion objective after adding one or two drops of liquid paraffin to the smears.

C. FAECAL EXAMINATION

(1) Direct method

One or two loopfuls of the faecal matter is mixed with water on a slide. A loopful of the diluted sample is then covered with a cover slip and examined under low and high power objectives of the microscope. This method is very useful in diagnosing coccidiosis in the fowls. Duodenal or caecal blood tinged scrappings can be used to detect coccidia. Suspended oocysts, merozoites and developmental stages of coccidia in the epithelial cells are noticed in direct wet mount preparations of intestinal mucosal scrappings of the infected birds.

(2) Concentration methods

(a) Sedimentation technique

The faecal sample is mixed with water and centrifuged. After discarding the supernatant, a loopful of the sediment is taken on to a slide and covered with a cover slip to examine the sediment under low and high powers.

(b) Floatation technique

(1) 2 to 3 gm of the faecal samples are liquified and sieved to remove the coarse particles.

(2) The liquified sample is poured into a centrifuge tube and centrifuged for 2 to 3 minutes at 1000 to 1500 rpm.

(3) The tube is taken out and the supernatant fluid is discarded and tube is filled with sugar solution. The sugar solution is prepared by dissolving 1 lb of sugar in 12 ounces of water under heat. A few drops of phenol (1% in water) is added to it to act like a preservative.

(4) The sugar solution and the sediment in a centrifuge tube is mixed by inverting the tube twice or thrice or then the tube is again centrifuged for 3 to 5 minutes.

(5) A drop of the supernatant fluid containing floating ova is

taken on a slide and covered with a cover glass. The preparation is then examined under low and high powers to detect ova or eggs of the parasites.

D. POULTRY FEED FORMULAE FOR PREPARING 100 KG OF FEEDS

A Feed formulae for birds

Ingredients	Starters (0-8 weeks) %	Growers (9-20 weeks) %	Layers (from 21 weeks onwards) %
Maize	52.00	50.00	50.00
Wheat bran	-	11.00	-
Rice polish	10.00	20.00	16.00
Groundnut extraction	14.00	9.00	20.00
Sun flower extraction	10.00	-	-
Fish meal	11.00	6.00	6.00
Shell grit	1.00	1.00	5.00
Bone meal	1.00	2.00	2.00
Nacl (common salt)	0 5	0.5	0.5
Mineral mixture	0.1	0.1	0.1
Vitamins	0.4	0.4	0.4

B. Feed formulae for broilers (aged about seven weeks)

Ingredients	Broilers starter (0-5 weeks)	Broilers finisher (6-8 weeks)
Maize	45.65	46.70
Rice polish	10.00	20.00
Groundnut cake	30.00	19.00
Fishmeal	13.00	13.00
Bone meal	0.75	0.70
Salt (Nacl)	0.40	0.40
Vitamins and mineral mixture	0.10	0.10
Furazolidone (Neftin) Coccidiostat	0.05	0.05
(Amprolium plus)	0.05	0.05

SOME NORMAL VALUES

Birds	Heart rate	Temperature
Fowls	350-470	105-110
Turkeys	200-280	104-106
Goose	200	105-107
Quails	500-600	-

E. SOME COMMON PRESERVATIVES

These are as follows :

	Preservatives	Specimens
1.	10% Formalin saline solution	1(a) Faeces emulsified in 10% formol saline for despatch to a diagnotic laboratory
2.	Formal saline solution 40% Formaldehyde 10 ml Sodium chloride Water	(b) Pieces of tissues (two cm cubed or 3-5mm thickness) are preserved in 10% formal saline solution 0.85 g 90 ml
3.	3 to 5% glycerine in 70% alcohol	(ii) Nematodes (preserved in 70% hot alcohol) containing 3-5% glycerin
4.	Absolute alcohol	(iii) Pieces of tissues for preserving the glycogen in the tissues

Note

The parasites are washed in normal saline before their preservation in hot 70% alcohol for fixation. Tapeworms are washed in saline solution (0.85% sodium chloride) before fixation for a few hours in 1-2% formal saline and these are then preserved in 70% alcohol for examination. Flukes are washed by shaking in saline solution in a test tube and these parasites (lightly pressed between slides) are then placed in a fixative(e.g. saturated aqueous solution of picrid acid 50 ml, distilled water 40 ml and glacial acetic acid 2 ml) for some time till opaque. These flukes are washed in tape water and processed through graded alcohols of different strengths (e.g. 70%, 80%, 90% and absolute alcohol) before being cleared in cresote for microscopic examination.

F. TABLE 17. SOME USEFUL INSECTICIDES (for eradicating the ectoparasites)

1.Parasites	2. Insecticide concentration	3. How to apply
Lice	Carbaryl 5% Fenchlorphos 0.05% Trichlorfon 0.15% Sodium fluoride 0.75% Derris 0.2%	To birds Spray on birds To birds as light spray Dip birds Dip birds
Poultry	Diazinon 0.5%	To birds
Redmite	Maldison 0.18%	To birds
Scaly leg mite	Sulphur Ointment 10%	Smear on legs
Fowl tick	Maldison 0.4-0.8% Diazinon 10%	Spray on birds to sheds
Stickfast	Maldison 5%	To birds
Flea	Derris 0.2%	Dip combs and wattles
Lice, ticks, mites and fleas	Cypermethrin, (Tick out)1ml/L	Spray on birds
Do	Aftox 50ml/L	To sheds, roof, floor and walls

Note : The birds are unsafe for human consumption until three days after treatment.

G. EXAMINATION OF ECTOPARASITES AND FUNGI ETC

a. Mites (the causative factors of cutaneous infestation or mange)

Insects, ticks and mites etc. are carriers of many pathogenic viruses, protozoa and spirochaetes etc in birds. Mites causing cutaneous lesions are noticed in the skin lesions or crushed nodules under a cover slip in one or two drops of acidulated water. Air-sac mites(*Cytoleichus spp.)* are detected in the air sacs and respiratory tract of the affected birds. Mange mites of the genus *Cnemidocoptes* are parasitic for only birds. Skin scrappings collected from the edge of active lesions are boiled gently for 5 minutes in 5 percent KOH solution and then centrifuged at 1500 r.p.m for about 5 to 10 minutes. The deposits are examined under low and high powers to detect the mites.

b. Some ectoparasites are seen in the internal organs of birds at autopsy.

c. Examination of fungi (mycotic agents)

Fungi(dermatophytes) are noticed in the scabs, crusts or epithelial cells in the cutaneous lesions. The crusts or epithelial cells in the lesions are placed on a slide in 10 to 40% solution of sodium or potassium hydroxide for microscopic examination under the low and high power objectives. *Trichophyton gallinae* (the causative agent of favus in chickens and turkeys) are found in the epidermal cells of scrappings. Interwoven hyphae with arthrospores are found in the the scabs or lesions of comb or scaly lesions on the different parts of the body of infected birds.

H. AVIAN AUTOPSY TECHNIQUE (RUBARTH, 1964)

Requirements

These are :

1. Scissors, knife, scalpel, forceps, sterile syringes, needles, vials, Petri dischaes, bone tongs (bone shears), wax pencil and glass slides etc.
2. Small autopsy table, small autoclave, instrument boiler, metal trays, respiratory mask, apron, hand gloves and gumboot etc.

Procedure

The legs are abducted by cutting or breaking open the hip joints. The abdomen is opened and the sternum is freed by lateral incisions through the ribs. The crop is then freed by blunt dissection from its attachment along the thoracic aperture to avoid being damaged when the heavy anterior osseous attachment of the sternum (the coracoid and clavicle) are clipped through with bone tongs on each side to join the lateral incisions through the ribs.

The liver is removed separately, avoiding damage to the gall bladder.

The spleen is removed separately

The stomach and intestinal canal are moved in one piece after cutting through the oesophagus just anterior to the proventriculus.

In sexually-mature females, the ovary is removed at its base and the oviduct is first extended by cutting through its dorsal and ventral mesenteric attachments and then removed by cutting through the cloaca.

The paricardial sac is incised and the chambers of the heart are opened in situ by incising the wall of the right ventricle near the apex and continuing the incision anteriorly up through the pulmonary artery and laterally up through the right atrium. The procedure is repeated for the left ventricle extending an incision at the apex up through the aorta and up through the left atrium. The heart is then removed by cutting through its base.

The lungs are freed by blunt dissection from thoracic walls, cutting through the dorsal attachment (dorsal to the thoracic oesophagus and aorta), and then removed by cutting through the trachea immediately anterior to the syrinx.

The upper beak is cut transversely at its base to expose the nasal cavities, and then the mouth is opened by cutting through one corner (the right is most convenient) and the incision continued through the pharynx and down the oesophagus to open the crop. The trachea is then opened along its whole length.

The brachial plexus and the sciatic nerve are exposed on both sides.

The major joints are opened.

Precautions

1. Inhalation of contaminated dust with infectious agents of communicable diseases (e.g. ornithosis or bird flu) should be avoided by wearing respiratory mask.

2. The intestines of the dead birds should be laid out on the table top for examination of lesions or parasites etc. as a last step after finishing the work of collecting the specimens for bacterial or viral isolation etc.
3. Sciatic nerve is examined by cutting the musculture on the medial side of the thigh for noticing the lesions of Marek's disease (MD).
4. The costochondral junctions are examined to observe enlargements (beadings). In cases of avian rickets, the bones are easily cut or bent without breaking.
5. The carcasses of birds should be incinerated (burnt up) or autoclaved to avoid infection to humans and healthy flocks of poultry and should never be thrown in the fields, ponds and rivers etc. to prevent infection to healthy birds.
6. Only systematic autopsy leads to a correct diagnosis of avian diseases.

1. Red and white blood cells count

The technique for counting avian blood cells differs from that of mammalian blood cell count because of nucleated red cells in birds. Nucleated red cells may be confused with lymphocytes.

White cell count

1. The semidirect Wiseman's method is quite suitable for counting of leucocytes. This diluent intensifies the eosinophilic cells in the chamber of haemocytometer and the percentage of these cells figured of the total WBC count of differential from a smear, the dilution plus the cells counted plus the percentages obtained allow total WBC value to be estimated.
2. The direct method involves use of a red cell pipette and a WBC diluent which stains the white cells and makes them to be distinguished from the red cells in the counting

chamber. This method allows direct counting of WBC. Count all the granulocytes in nine large squares . Divide the number of leucocytes counted by 9 to obtain the value of leucocytes per square mm. Then, the total number of leucocytes per cubic millimeter of blood is calculated considering the dilution factor of the blood and the thickness (0.1mm) of blood sheet on the haemocytometer. For example, if the dilution factor for the blood is one in 200 and the total number of white cells in one central and 4 corner squares is X, then the total number of white cells per cubic mm of the blood is 10,000 X.

Diluent for semidirect method (Wiseman's method)

1. Wiseman's fluid
Phloxine 50 mg
Formalin (40% formaldehyde) 5ml
Ringer's solution 95ml

2. Ringer's solution
Sodium chloride 0.7g
Sodium bicarbonate 0.03 g.
Potassium chloride 0.026 g.
Calcium chloride 0.003 g.
Distilled water 1000 ml

Procedure

A. Red cell count

Fill the red cell pipette up to 0.5 mark with avian blood and fill rest of the pipette to the 101 mark with Wiseman's fluid. One hour of gentle agitation is best for maximum staining of eosinophilic cells containing acidophilic granules. These are easily counted in the haemocytometer. Count all the nucleated red cells in 80 of the small squares (i.e. one central and 4 corner squares). If the dilution factor for the blood is 1 in 200, the total red cell count in one central and 4 corner squares is multiplied by 10,000 to estimate the red cell count per cubic millimeter of the undiluted blood.

B. White cell count

Wiseman's diluent highly intensifies the acidophilic granules of heterophils. All the acidophilic granulocytes in the entire ruled area of the haemocytometer are counted. A differential count of white cells of the blood in question is performed to obtain the proportionate values of heterophils, lymphyocytes, monocytes and basophils.Then, the value of white cells per cubic millimeter is calculated by the process of semidirect method as indicated above.

Diluent for direct method

Blain solution 1

Neutral red 1 part

Lockeds solution 5,000 parts

(adjusted to PH 7.4)

Blain solution 2

Formalin 12%

Lockeds solution 88%

(adjusted to pH 7.4)

Procedure (direct method for white cell count)

Fill the rbc pipette up to the 0.5 mark with blood, take solution 1 until half of the bulb is filled and then finish filling of the pipette up to the 101mark with solution II.The white cells in the blood are stained by the diluent no1 and are easily differentiated from the red cells in the counting chamber. The rest of the procedure for counting leucocytes is similar to one as followed in the case of mammalian blood.

J. RAPID METHOD FOR STAINING SPIROCHAETES.

1. Prepare thin blood smears on the clean glass slides.
2. Fix the smears on the glass slides by dipping the slides in a wide mouth bottle containing methyl alcohol and leave them in methyl alcohol for 5 minutes.
3. Stain with 0.5% aqueous crystal violet for 20 seconds.
4. Wash these slides with tap water.
5. Blot them dry with blotting paper and examine the stained

smears under oil immersion objective after taking one or two drops of liquid paraffin over the smear.

The spirochaetes stain deep purple and the red cells stain high colour.

K. NORMAL RANGE OF BLOOD VALUES OF POULTRY

RBC (millions)	2.8-4.5
WBC (thousands)	20-40
Heterophils (percent)	31 (20 - 40)
Basophils (percent)	1.4 (2-5)
Eosinophils (percent)	6 (2-10)
Lymphocytes (percent)	78 (55-96)
Monocytes (percent)	1 (0-3)
Haemoglobin grams per 100 ml	8.0 - 13.0

Blood picture of chickens

Cells	Male	Female
Red cells	3,230,000	2,720,000
Thrombocytes	25,400	26,500
Leucocytes	19,800	19,800
Differential %	-	-
Lymphocytes	59.1	64.61
Heterophils	27.2	22.8
Eosinophils	01.9	01.9
Basophils	1.7	1.7
Monocytes	10.2	8.9
Haemoglobin%	11.76	9.1

L. DISEASES OF ZOO, WILD AND SOME LABORATORY ANIMALS

Zoological pathology deals with diseases of invertebrates, fish, amphibions, reptiles, birds and mammals. Knowledge on pathology of diseases of dometic animals and birds makes a better understanding of diseases of wild animals and birds in captivity. Basically ,the lesions and signs of a disease (say, a bacterial or a viral infection in domestic animals) do not differ from those in wild or zoo animals .

Information on wild life in captivity needs a deep study of diseases of zoo animals. Many infectious diseases of captive animals have high communicability and pathogenicity for animals and man. A brief description of diseases and their causes of zoo and laboratory animals has been given in Table-18.

Table 18 . Some of the diseases of captive animals

Diseases	Causes	Hosts
1. African horse sickness	An Orbivirus	Equidae, dog
2. African swine fever	An Iridovirus	Suidae
3. Borna disease	Virus-unclassified	Equidae and bovidae
4. Epizootic lymphangitis	*Histoplasma farciminosus*	Equidae
5. Contagious bovine pleuropneumonia	*Mycoplasma mycoides var mycoides*	Cattle, yak, antelope, buffalo, bison and reindeer
6.Eastcoast fever	*Theileria parva*	Cattle and African Buffalo
7. Bovine ephemeral fever	Rhabdovirus	Cattle
8. Foot and Mouth disease	Rhinovirus	All artiodactyla
9. Fowl Plague/ Avian influenza	An Orthomyxovirus	All aves

Diseases	Causes	Hosts
10.Glanders	*Pseudomonas mallei*	Equidae and Carnivora
11.Dourine	*Trypanosoma equiperdum*	Equidae
12. Heart water	*Cowdria ruminantium*	Bovidae
13. Haemorrhagic septicaemia	Pasteurella multocida (Type B)	Cattle and buffalo.
14. Japanese encephalitis	Flarivirus	Equidae, Suedae and man
5. Louping ill	Flarivirus	Cattle, sheep, shrew, man, wood mouse and red grouse
16. Nairobi sheep disease	Bunyavirida (ungrouped)	Sheep and goats
17. Peste-des-petits ruminants(PPR)	Paramyxovirus(PPR virus,a morbillivirus closely related to the RP virus)	Sheep and goats
18. Rift valley fever	Bunyaviridae (ungrouped)	Bovidae, suidae and man
19. Rinderpest	Paramyxovirus	Most Artiodactyla
20. Sheep Pox	Pox virus	Sheep
21. Sweating sickness	Tick born toxicosis	Cattle
22. Swine vesicular disease	Enterovirus, porcine, Coxackie 1	Suidae
23. Teschen Diseased	Enterovirus, porcine 1	Suidae
24. Venezuelan equine encephalomyelitis	Alpha virus	Equidae and Canidae
25. Viscerotropic-Velogenic Newcastle Disease	Paramyxovirus	Poultry and wild birds
26. Hogcholera	Togavirus	Suidae

Other reportable diseases in captive animals are anaplasmosis, anthrax, blue tongue, brucellosis, babesiosis, (cattle tick fever), equine babesiosis, leptospirosis, psroptic cattle scabies, equine encephalomyelitis, fowl typhoid, infectious laryngotracheitis, pullorum disease, mammalian tuberculosis, equine infections anaemia, rabies, salmonellosis, vesicular stomatitis, bovine mammillitis, duck viral hepatitis and psittacosis.

Metabolic bone diseases, osteoporosis, osteomalacia, rickets, hyperthyroidism and osteodystrophia fibrosa are also noticed in wild animals

Infections stomatitis is noticed in snakes. Abscesses are frequently noticed in reptitles. Fungal dermatitis has been reported in a desert tortoise. The viruses causing eastern, western and Japanese B encephalitis have been found in reptiles.

Penguins, cranes, storks and flamingoes are important zoo birds.

Trematodes, cestodes, nematodes and arthropods are noticed in birds. Intestinal coccidiosis is an important disease in birds. Sarcocystis spp. has been reported from raptors. Diabetes mellitus is reported in birds. Rabies is also recorded in nonhuman primates and wild mammals.

Tuberculosis is an important disease affecting non-human primates and deers etc.

Some important carnivores in zoo are as under:

Families	**Animals**
Canidae	Dogs, foxes, and wolves
Ursidae	Bears
Procyonidae	Raccoon, kinkajou and panda
Mustelidae	Skunks, otter and weasel
Viverridae	Civets and mongoose
Hyaenidae	Hyenas
Felidae	Cats

Ascarids (roundworms), hookworms, wheepworms, stomachworms, tapeworms, flukes, thornyheaded worms, lungworms, heartworms and pinworms also infect wild carnivores. Important wild felids (family Felidae) include felines like ocelot, margay, pampascat, sandcat, pellascat, senvalcat, lynx, bobcat, coracol, European wild cat, mountain lion, clouded leopard, snow leopard, leopard, jaguar, lion, tiger and cheetah. Deficiencies of iron, iodine, copper, manganese, zinc, vitamin 'A' and vitamin 'E' are known diseases in felines. Viral rhinotracheitis, calcivirus infection, reovirus infection and pneumonitis in felines have been reported. Intranuclear inclusion bodies and intracytoplasmic inclusion bodies are found in feline viral rhinotracheitis (FVR) and feline pneumonitis (FPN) respectively. Wild felids also suffer from ascaridiasis, hookworms, stomachworms and tapeworms etc. The important canids amongst wild animals are timber wolf, Indian wolf, blackbacked jackal, Asiatic jackal, hunting dog, bush dog, kit fox, cape fox, gray fox, arctic fox, fennec fox, bat-eared fox, maned fox and raccoon dogs etc.

Elephants are the largest living land animals. Bull African elephants reach a height of 3.6 m at the shoulder and weigh about 6400 kg. Anthrax, salmonellosis, tuberculosis, clostridial diseases (enterotoxaemias), colibacillosis, pasteurella infection (haemorrhagic septicaemia) etc are reported in elephants. Elephant pox and herpes virus infection of the lungs are important viral diseases of elephants. Elephants also suffer from sun burn, rash, dermatitis and traumatic injuries in wild state.

Skin ulceration and neoplasms like fibromas are also reported in elephants. Subcutaneous oedema as large pockets of oedematous sole, cracked sole, cracked heal and overgrown sole and over grown nails are other pathological conditions of elephants. Overgrowth of cuticle, wounds, abscessation, laminitis, fractures, dislocations and degenerative joint diseases are seen in elephants. Elephants also die of volvulus, intussusception and choke etc. These animals are susceptible to heat stroke and frost bites. Protozoa like *Trypanosoma* spp. and *Babaesia* spp. infect elephants. Trematodes and several species of filarids are also noticed in the affected elephants . Obstructions of small intestine with ascarids are reported in equidae(zebras).

Important artiodactylids are Suidae (pigs), Tayassuidae (peccaries),Hippopotamidae(hippos), Camelidae (camels and llamas), cervidae (deers), Giraffidae (Giraffe and okapi), Antilocapridae (pronghorn) and Bovidae (antelope, wild cattle, goats and sheep). Johne's disease is noticed in wild cattle, sheep and goats and is marked by infectious enteritis. Blue tongue is seen in domestic and wild ruminants. Malignant catarrhal fever is an important disease of wild ruminants. Important internal parasites of artiodactylids are *Pneumostronglyus, Protostronglyus, Echnicoccus, Taenia, Fasciola, Elaephora, Haemonchus, Ostertagia, Trichostrongylus, Cooperia, Bunostomum, Strongloides, Chabertia, Ascaris, Nematodirus, Trichuria, Eimeria, Toxoplasma, Trichinelle, Sarcocystis, Babesia, Theileria* and *Trypanosoma* etc.

Tigers

Panleukopenia (feline distemper) is reported in leopards, lions and tigers, Salmonellosis, anthrax and tuberculosis are diseases which have been noticed in felines. T B has been seen in Siberian tigers. Surra caused by *Trypanosoma evansi* is an important disease affecting tigers. *Babesia felis* is reported to infect lions. Zoo felids also suffer from toxoplasmosis. Coccidiosis is an important disease of zoo felines.

Important lagomorphes and rodents kept in zoo are as follows:

(1) Family Leporidae (rabbit and hare),

(2) Sciuromorpha (squirrels, marmuts, gophers)

(3) Myomorpha (rats mice, hamsters, lemmings and voles).

Vultures

Vultures (natural scavengers like white backed, long billed and slender billed) contribute to the cleanliness of the environment and prevent spread of diseases by disposing of the carcasses of animals (say, adult cattle being consumed by vultures in about 20 minutes). They are facing extinction due to drooping neck syndrome caused by use of the veterinary drug 'diclofenac' in treating sick animals .

The diseases reported in rodents are plague (*Yersinia* pestis infection), pasteurellosis (*Pasteurella multocida* infection), listeriosis (*Listeria monocytogenes* infection), viral encephalitis (EEE, WEE and VEE) and coccidioidomycosis. Many species of rodents are susceptible to rabies. Dermatophytes frequently infect the rodents. Guinea pig is very susceptible to tuberculosis. Rodents are susceptible to trematodes and cestodes. Cases of toxoplasmosis, babesiosis, trypanosomiasis, Leishmaniasis, coccidiosis and giardiasis are also known to occur in rodents. Symptoms and pathological lesions noticed in domestic diseased birds and animals are important bases to understand the disease processes of their counterparts in captivity. Moreover, it is the wild animals which are the sources of the domestic animals kept by human beings and animate infectious agents attack both groups of animals (i.e. the wild and domestic animals).

References

1. Calnek, B.W (1991) Diseases of poultry, 9th edition, Iowa State University Press, Iowa
2. Chu. H.P (1960) A laboratory handbook on diagnosis of poultry diseases. Animal health branch monograph No. 2. F.A.O. Rome.
3. Fowler, Murray E (1978) Zoo and wild animal medicine, W.B. Saunders Sompany Philadelphia, London and Toronto.
4. Fowler, Murray E (1993) Zoo and wild animal medicine, W.B. Saunders Company Philadelphia, London and Toronto.
5. Mall, B.K. (1995) Personal communication. Farm Vet. Officer A.H. Department, Bihar.

INDEX